Spa Manicuring for the Salon and Spa

Janet McCormick

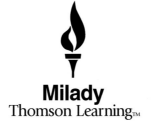

Milady
Thomson Learning™

Africa • Australia • Canada • Denmark • Japan • Mexico • New Zealand • Philippines
Puerto Rico • Singapore • Spain • United Kingdom • United States

NOTICE TO THE READER

Milady Staff:

Milady President: Susan L. Simpfenderfer

Executive Editor: Marlene McHugh-Pratt

Acquisitions Editor: Pamela Lappies

Developmental Editor: Judy Roberts

Executive Production Manager: Wendy Troeger

Production Editor: Suzanne Nelson

Executive Marketing Manager: Donna Lewis

Channel Manager: Nigar Hale

Channel Manager: Eleanor J. Murray

Cover Design: Cathleen Berry/TerraLuma Design

Online Services

Milady Online
To access a wide variety of Milady products and services on the World Wide Web, point your browser to:
http://www.milady.com

Delmar Online
To access a wide variety of Delmar products and services on the World Wide Web, point your browser to:
http://www.delmar.com
or email: info@delmar.com

Library of Congress Cataloging-in-Publication Data

McCormick, Janet
       Spa manicuring for the salon and spa / by Janet McCormick.
          p.   cm.
       ISBN: 1-56253-460-2
       1.Manicuring. 2. Nails (Anatomy)—Care and hygiene. 3. Hand—Massage. I. Title.
TT958.3 .M33 1999   99-046252
646.7'27— dc21   CIP

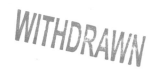

TABLE OF CONTENTS

PREFACE

Spa Manicuring for the Salon and Spa is written to for you, the career professionals who wish to improve and upgrade your work and our industry. You are the future through whom our industry will be expanded. Others will learn through your example, and the industry will grow.

The goal of this book is to aid you in expanding your knowledge and skills in manicuring and, therefore, your success. The new information can take your manicuring skills into the Millennium and provide you with an entirely new view of the nail industry. You can, if you wish, become a "full service" manicurist, allowing you to provide the best service possible for a client, no matter their needs.

This book has been set up as a background information first, procedures second, then in-salon implementation procedures last. I hope you will read the information and set forth with the skills in that order as it will provide a deeper, more lasting internalization into your professional life.

The procedures have been tested for you at the table by excellent professional technicians. These technicians truly care about their work, and believe that others within their profession will be interested in improving their table effectiveness through these methods. These procedures are not written in stone, however. They are a base, a foundation for your own creativeness. As professionals you can start from here and create your own unique and beautiful style. The wealth of creativity you can develop from this information is the beauty of spa manicuring.

Particularly important to the results you will see in using these skills are the products you will introduce into the services. Each description of a skill will describe specific ingredients needed in the products to achieve the desired results. To achieve these results, it is important that you shop for, learn about, and practice with the best products you can purchase for use at your table and for retailing, according to the company's directions and within their restrictions.

If you like these procedures, I suggest that you begin to test and integrate the information immediately into your routine so that it will become part of your working knowledge. The sooner you use and apply them, the more "spa" you will be!

ACKNOWLEDGMENTS

A special thank you to the following people and organizations for contributing to this book. The author appreciates their efforts toward the final product of *Spa Manicuring*.

Editors and staff of Milady Publishing Company.

Sue Ellen Schultes, Notorious Nails, Green Brook, New Jersey, for her assistance with the photo program and text review. Also Kimberley Comisky and Lori Murillo of Kimberley's Day Spa for their professionalism, talent, and accommodation.

My twin sister, Jane Seiling, Lima, Ohio, and my twin daughters, both nail techs, Dawn McCormick, Columbus, Ohio, and Denise Baich, Balwin Missouri, who pushed me into finishing when I became discouraged.

My favorite editor, my sister, Jackie Muter, Director of Windward Island School of Evangelism, St. Vincent, West Indies, who helped me make it readable.

All the professionals who encouraged me to write this book because they felt it would make a positive contribution to professionalism and profits in our industry.

Vicki Peters of The Peters Perspective, Las Vegas, Nevada

Sheryl Macauley of Spaz—The Professional Nail Art System, Bakersfield, California

April Buford of Truman College, Chicago, Illinois

Ginny Burge of Beautique Day Spa and Salon, Houston, Texas

Grace Francis of Vista, California

Laura Manicho of Nationwide Beauty Academy, Amlin, Ohio

Florence Hogan of Avanti Salon, Sterling Heights, Michigan

LaCinda Headings of Xenon International School of Hair Design, Hutchinson, Kansas

Kathleen Matti-LaSalle of LeTresee Salon and Spa, Totowa, New Jersey

FOREWORD

By Linda W. Lewis

Having served as editor of both Nailpro and DAYSPA for several years, I'm in a position to know exactly how helpful the book you're holding in your hands is to manicurists, nail technicians, and salon owners. If you call yourself a manicurist, you probably already specialize in natural nail care and you may even use some of the techniques discussed herein. Nevertheless, you're sure to find additional tips that will help you serve your clients better, and to discover business and professional insights that will allow you to take your services (and your income) to a higher level.

Do manicures bring in the same amount of revenue as other services in your salon that require the same amount of time and expertise? How can you command higher prices for your manicures? Do you know why waterless manicures are better for your clients' nails? Do you know when to make exceptions and provide water soaks? Do you have to work in a day spa to offer spa services? How can you protect yourself and your clients from transmissible diseases in the salon? Do you know what causes age spots and how you can help your clients minimize them? How can you get the respect you deserve from salon owners, co-workers and clients? You'll find thorough and interesting discussions of each of these questions in Spa Manicuring for the Salon and Spa.

If you call yourself a nail technician and specialize in nail enhancements, you need to consider the current trend toward natural nail care. With the general emphasis on pure and natural in all the products we use, many clients who once wore acrylics or fiberglass wraps are now looking for new solutions to their nail problems. This book includes the information you need to add natural nail care services to your salon menu and offers suggestions that will make your new services both exciting and profitable.

How can you make as much money doing manicures as you did with nail enhancements? Can waterless manicure techniques be used with clients who wear nail enhancements without causing lifting? How can you analyze each client's hands and nails and prescribe appropriate salon services and at-home care? Answers to these questions, as well as the ones above, will make your transition to natural nail care easier and more profitable.

During 25 years as the editor of various special interest publications, it has been my job to discover knowledgeable people in particular professions and work with them to convey their considerable expertise to others in their field. Finding a true expert who can effectively communicate his or her special techniques and insights is rare; Janet McCormick is one of the few I have met in my career. Not only does she know her subject matter—how to care for nails and hands and how to run a successful salon—but she has a gift for communicating the lessons she has learned from constant training and years of experience to anyone willing to learn. No matter where you are in the nail profession, you're sure to find this work both insightful and inspiring. Over the years we've worked together, Janet has written dozens of articles for both Nailpro and DAYSPA. Often she suggests article ideas that would never have occurred to me, imparting detailed information that only she and few other expertly trained and highly experienced nail technicians would know. This deep understanding of her subject matter is combined with an organized mind and a command of the English language that lets her convey both general and specific instruction in easily understood form. She continues to teach me something new with nearly every article she writes. I'm sure you'll enjoy Spa Manicuring for the Salon and Spa as much as I have.

INTRODUCTION: ARE MANICURES FOR ME?

After 2000+ years of existence, manicuring nearly died a quick death with the establishment of wearable enhancements. We technicians were certain that every woman would wear them and that manicuring was an outmoded skill that would probably disappear. Movie stars and the media agreed with us. Cher wore them long and square on her TV variety show, and Dan Rather stated in a segment of his television news magazine that was shown the year I opened my first salon (1980), "It's estimated that 80% of the women will be wearing artificial nails by the year 2000." I was thrilled and went to work happy the next day! I had focused my nails-only salon on acrylic nails and not on the boring manicures I had learned in beauty school.

Although enhancements improved quickly after their development, manicures had not changed much or improved over their thousands of years of existence. They continued to be what they were at their inception: soak, push back the cuticles, and so on. If the consumer watched "Madge" on her TV commercial, she felt quite capable of doing her own nails, and as professionals, we were not doing much to change her opinion of this service.

Because we were trained as manicurists, we did manicures in my salon, when we could not avoid them. However, when we did one, the clients returned for another! After a manicure, the client's nails, cuticles, and skin were nearly the same as when they came in, just cleaned up a bit and coated with fresh polish. Every week we would hope to see some significant improvement in the client's nails as a result of our work, but it rarely happened. Manicures were frustrating for us to do, and our work gave few reasons for the clients to return to us repeatedly.

Manicures were boring in 1980. No new products were appearing that would improve the service and our results, and the products and techniques were the same as they were in the 1930's. Most nail manufacturers were not interested in developing new products for this skill. More profit could be made in

acrylic products at that time, and consumers were more interested in artificial nails than in manicures. In addition, little education was available to enhance our skills on natural nail services, so we were fast losing interest in doing them. Who wants to do a service that's a frustrating routine? No wonder that we tried to put every client into enhancements!

As we upgraded our skills and titles to 'nail technician' and enjoyed the resulting creativity acrylics allowed, many of us left manicures behind or we avoided them totally. I remember the receptionist sneaking manicures onto our books. I'd say, "I have a manicure next...ugh!" when I saw them on the book. And I was the owner!

We did them begrudgingly...and poorly, probably. We wanted to be known as nail technicians, not manicurists, so we passed them to the "newbies"— who passed them on to newer technicians as soon as their appointment books were filled with acrylics. Or we put our creative brains aside when we could not avoid doing them.

We disliked doing manicures for good reason. We could offer only two services, the "basic manicure," which was a water-soak manicure, and the "hot oil manicure," which was the heated lotion soak manicure. Neither improved the client's nails. Later, we added the heated mitts and a paraffin dip as added-value treatments for the cuticles and skin, but only rarely did we suggest them as a service for our clients. We wanted to do acrylics!

Enhancements made us more money, they were fun to do, and our clients thought they were miraculous; we looked like angels of mercy to our clients. Arriving, they hated their nails; leaving, they loved them and showed them off proudly. They paid for them happily and were programmed to return on a regular basis, while the client with natural nails could grow discouraged and drop off the client list altogether.

Spa Manicuring for the Salon and Spa

Goodbye to the "Basic" and "Hot Oil"

The situation has changed in recent years. Manicuring is becoming a more popular service, to the dismay of many nail technicians and to the delight of a few. The "Baby Boomers" have learned about skin care, with its ability to help them look and feel younger, and their hands are now included in their concerns. They are becoming educated and are desperately seeking that special manicurist who is willing to go that extra mile to produce impressive results...immediately, if possible. When she is discovered, her clients tell their friends and her books are filled. She is as popular as any enhancement technician, and as rewarded.

Luckily, manicurists now have the potential to meet demands by their clients for healthy and beautiful nails and skin; products have become available to help us produce impressive results. At first most products were from the skin care industry. When a manicurist would stumble onto skin care products that produced great results in her manicures, the revelation was one of those "Ah-haaaa!" reactions: the products were there, but we had not known about them. They were being used for skin care only, until we found them. We discovered that with a few technique modifications, they worked for our clients, too! We would incorporate these products into manicures that made these new and loyal clients happy.

Now, new products are being regularly released to us from within our industry—products that help us perform the miracles our clients want for their hands. Even the nail enhancement companies are beginning to produce great manicuring products, some with skin care-oriented professional and retail regimens, after all those years of ignoring manicuring as uninteresting and unprofitable. They are delighted with the successful and profitable expansion of their product lines into care of the hands, and so are we, their customers.

We are introducing these new products into services for out clients' hands and see dramatic results on very happy clients. A new kind of skill has been introduced by these products: skin care-oriented manicures. Those of us educated in skin care of the hands are excited about our new capabilities for meeting the needs of our clients. We are stepping beyond the era of the water manicure, basic manicure, or hot oil manicure into a new niche of clients who are serious about the health and beauty of their entire hands, not just the beauty of their nail plates.

Will the Enhancement Stay On If We Do Skin Care?

An immediate concern of the technicians who do enhancements is the effects of skin care treatments on the adhesion of the client's acrylics. Be assured that skin care treatments can be incorporated into an enhancement technician's services without harming or causing the enhancement to lift.

The taboo of using any oil on the skin and nails during the application appointment for enhancements has been replaced with "apply oil to the cuticles" and "apply oil to the enhancement." The product lines use abundant oils during their techniques now; the forbidden use of oils is old news. Oils are now allowed because:

They are essential oils with tiny molecules that are absorbed into the skin quickly, even as they "plasticize" and moisturize the nail.

The enhancements, if preparation and application are correct, are not affected negatively by essential oils.

The oils act as a barrier on the surface of the acrylic, promoting a more speedy polymerization by the acrylic product.

When choosing the time to do a skin care treatment for a client who is wearing enhancements, the spa professional has several choices. Consider the following:

If a service is performed before the acrylic service, simple and effective preparation is performed before the application of the product with a thorough cleansing and correct preparation of the nail plate for the enhancement.

The service can be offered as a separate visit. Many clients enjoy a manicure/re-polish between enhancement appointments.

The treatment can be performed after the fill. The base coat is applied and allowed to dry, then the skin care treatment is done. After the treatment, the base coat is removed for some treatments, reapplied, and the polish step is completed. For other treatments, the polish can immediately be applied over the base coat.

Skin care treatments should not be blamed for lifting; assumptions that lotions and oils are the cause of lifting are incorrect and outdated. If lifting occurs, technicians should never say to the client, "I wonder if it's the oils." Instead, she should look at her preparation and application technique and her client's lifestyle.

The acrylic technicians are one step ahead when introducing skin care to their clients—their clients have already bought into having beautiful nails and have made a statement by their prior services that they are committed to beautiful hands. "Beautiful hands are the 'frame' around beautiful nails," a friend once said to me. "A beautiful picture needs a beautiful frame." These clients will easily accept the total picture—skin care for their hands will show off their beautiful nails perfectly! They need skin care treatments for beautifying the skin on their hands and will accept the treatments and home care readily—if they are introduced to them by their technician.

Skin care is always a benefit to a client, enhancing her technician's worth to her. The informed client with acrylic nails appreciates the new and improved appearance of her hands, arms, and elbows; purchases many home care products; and will likely come in for services more frequently. Her tickets and tips are higher because the appearance of her hands has improved. This book will help you discover how you can use these skills in a new age of manicuring.

Millennium Potential

Manicures and skin care treatments for the hands are fast becoming essential to a nail department meeting its millennium potential. The nail-table-in-the-corner and the professional who merely does nails are becoming a thing of the past. Such narrow service offerings may be a sign of poor expertise to some clients, whether that is an accurate assumption or not. In these instances, the professional will either suffer a lower income or will be forced to upgrade and broaden her skills.

The clients of Millennium 2000 are increasingly knowledgeable and are demanding more visual and therapeutic results in their beauty services, including their manicures. They know what they want, and great manicures that include treatments for beautifying their skin are it.

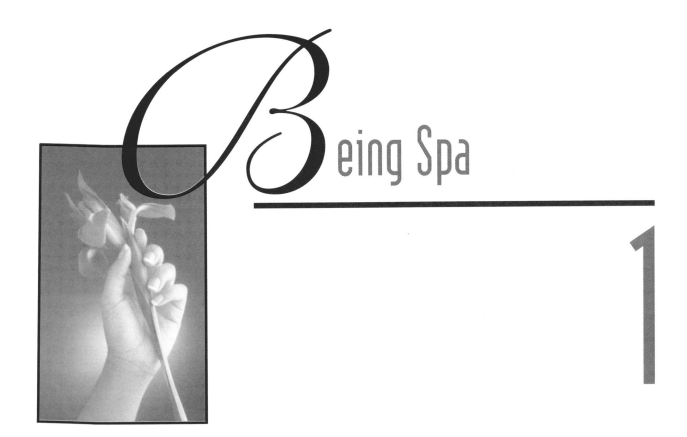

Being Spa

1

OBJECTIVES

At the end of this chapter, you should be able to:

- Define the concept of "spa."
- State that spa is not a "place."
- Describe how to become a spa.
- Define the importance of training in the spa concept.
- Describe the philosophy of analysis-driven manicures.
- State spa service concepts.
- Use spa concepts in routine decision-making processes.

According to Faith Popcorn, the guru of trends, day spas are the "wave of the future."

She suggests that due to time and money constraints on their lives, working men and women can not "recharge their batteries" with the conventional relaxation time. However, according to Popcorn, they can enjoy a relaxing time away from their stresses for renewal in a spa environment. Spas will become increasingly successful, Popcorn believes.

Spas survive or die around their ability to recharge their clients during every visit, whether in a full day or an hour. The services go beyond even the most professional and upscale salon in every way, and every aspect of a spa is focused on making the visit memorable for the client.

WHAT IS "SPA"?

Originally coined in Europe, "spa" is a term used to describe a certain type of salon and level of services. However, the American spa concept is different from the European concept because it focuses more on pampering and rejuvenation than in Europe where it may be a more medically driven industry. True American spa concept services are described in the following terms:

Quiet — This salon is not "rockin' and rollin'." The noise level is low and the music is subtle and calming, encouraging the client to relax, reflect, and revitalize. She immerses in the quiet. (Fig. 1–1)

Figure 1-1

The quiet elegance of the salon gives the client a warm, welcoming feeling.

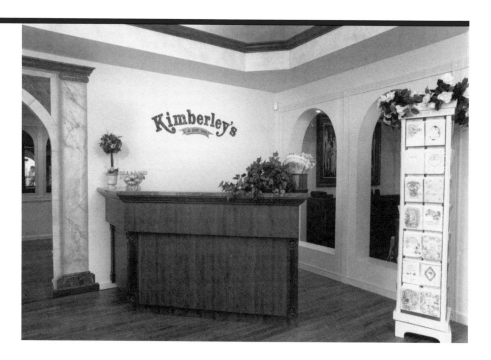

Spa Manicuring for the Salon and Spa

Clean—This salon is immaculate. The professionals and auxiliary personnel are all aware of the importance of cleanliness to their clients and are dedicated to producing a consistently clean environment for them.

Pampering—Clients are in this salon to be pampered; the first priority of the professionals and auxiliary personnel of these salons is to meet their wishes and needs.

Therapeutic—Clients arrive with the desire and expectation that they will feel better when they leave. The environment is designed to facilitate these feelings, and the services are designed to immediately make a difference for them.

Luxurious surroundings—The surroundings are beyond the environments of any of the salons these clients have patronized, though they are not necessarily more expensive. The luxury is designed to provide an overall perception of being pampered. (Fig. 1–2)

Separate—A spa is set apart from the noise and hubbub of the busy world and probably even from the more noisy areas of the rest of the salon. They can walk through the doors of these facilities and feel they are removed from stress. Watches are discouraged (or at least looking at them) while they are in this separate world.

Professional dress—The professionals dress according to a code, in congruence with the décor, each other, and the overall spa concept. (No bare midriffs here!)

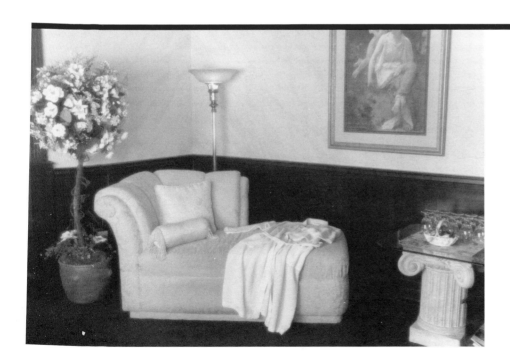

Figure 1-2

The luxurious surroundings give the perception of being pampered.

Aromatherapy—The spa area has aromas that are calming and enjoyable, uplifting and rejuvenating. Non-spa aromas are managed through ventilation and professional techniques.

Skilled professionals—Because these clients expect superior service, they also expect spa professionals who are highly skilled. The professionals are confident, informed, informative, caring, and dedicated to the concept of spa.

High-quality products—The clients can be confident that the products they purchase in a nail spa have been chosen for their superior ingredients and performance.

Ambiance—The surroundings in a spa concept salon support the relaxation, rejuvenation, and beautification that the client wishes to accomplish. Nothing unpleasant is allowed to assault her senses. The décor is usually thematic, and the environment is upscale.

Rejuvenating/calming—Spa clients justify their visits to a spa concept salon by the feeling of the renewal they achieve during their services. Their time in the spa atmosphere becomes their de-stressing time. (Fig. 1–3)

Focused—A spa is focused on the client and meeting her needs. Every skill, decision, and activity has this as its goal.

Figure 1-3

The client can indulge in her surroundings and relax stress-free.

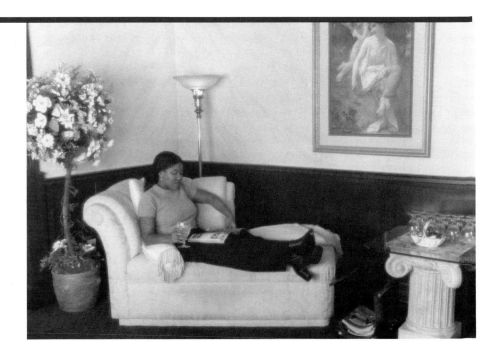

Spa Manicuring for the Salon and Spa

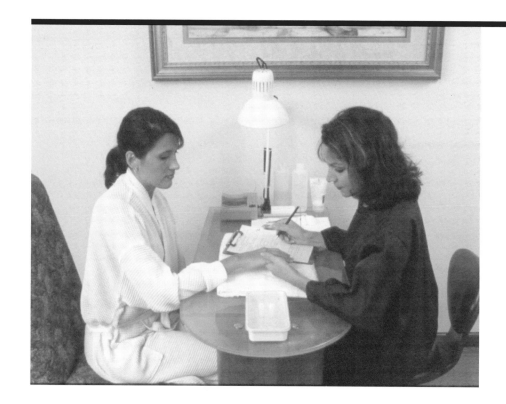

Figure 1-4

The client analysis is an integral aspect of spa manicuring.

Analysis driven — A client-focused salon will use analysis and consultation to determine the client's needs, recommend services, and home care products to meet these needs. (Fig. 1–4)

Consistent — Spas are consistent in very aspect of spa concept; the services are performed according to standard practices, the aromas are familiar and as expected, cleanliness is continually upheld — every aspect will have a planned sameness. The clients will know what to expect on their return visits, no matter which professional performs the service.

Higher in cost — The services in a spa concept salon are high quality and probably higher in cost; these clients are prepared to pay for them.

If the characteristics of spa concept can be summed up in a word by a client she might use *"specialness."* This word defines *a synergy of details that have been successfully planned and implemented to produce a feeling, a mind-set,* in the spa client during and after her visit. During the visit, she is quieter, more relaxed, more cooperative, "more everything" than she would be in a non-spa concept salon. Afterward, she conjures up special feelings about the salon and its professionals when she recalls the visit.

To produce this synergy, the spa concept salons/professionals must focus on successfully meeting the individual characteristics of spa concept, even the little details, through careful planning and implementation. If these are met, the client will feel her expenditures are worth it, will tell her friends, and return often.

Spa clients will more frequently express their pleasure or displeasure to the management and their friends. Many know what "spa" is and are less forgiving of the shortcomings of spa concept salons than of regular salons. They may say of a salon, "Oh well, a bad hair day;" this is not so of a spa visit. Spas must strive to the fullest to earn their higher fees or the client will not return and will discuss her disappointment with their friends.

Spa Concept: Not a <u>Place</u>

You say, "I'm not a spa." Or, "I don't work in a spa. What does all this have to do with me?" Spa is an *attitude*, not a *place*, though the surroundings should support its achievement. It is a *concept of client service*. Spa concept is an *orientation*, an *ambiance*, and an *awareness*, all provided for the client at a particular level of service. It is an *overarching professional philosophy* for the decision-making, activities, and professional developments within the salon. (It is not accomplished by adding "Day Spa" to a salon's name.)

Spa concept does not even have to be in a full-service salon, a spa, or an entire salon; it can be in a "nails only" salon in a neighborhood or within a specialty department in a salon. The clients will sense the difference and immediately respond to it.

A nail professional in a lease station within a non-spa salon can bring her room or area into spa concept, even considering her limitations within her non-spa surroundings. If she cannot provide a separate environment, she *can* incorporate spa treatments and services, changing what is within her power, despite the ambiance in the surroundings. These changes will set her apart from the traditional manicurists and acrylic artists with whom she is competing. They will even set her apart from the other technicians within the salon where she works, if she wishes to do so. (Fig. 1–5)

The spa treatments and manicures a spa professional provides will enhance her importance in the life of her clients. She enjoys the heightened loyalty and respect she will be given by clients who like the results they enjoy and for their manicurist to be a step ahead of their friend's. They reward her with higher tickets and referrals, resulting in her possessing a confidence and professionalism that she's never before enjoyed.

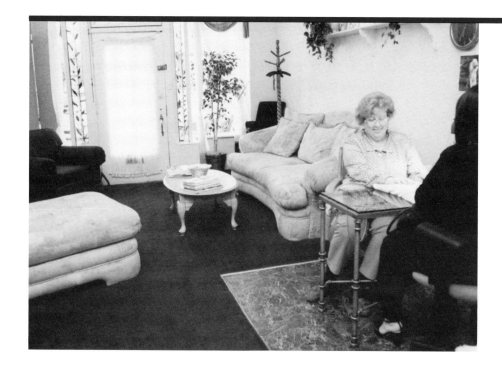

Figure 1-5

A separate room and environment will set a manicurist apart from the competition.

Becoming "Spa" Starts with Training

A nail salon, department, or a single table can become spa by incorporating spa service concepts within the service orientation and the services, perhaps even more so than many real spas. However, knowledge and confidence are needed to succeed. It all begins with a training process and requires continual retraining.

As spa treatments and manicures are being developed, the technical training programs for their use are being developed also. However, salon-owners can embrace the concept and train personnel, but the responsibility for success ultimately resides with the individual spa professional's dedication to the details of spa concept. This salon will have the vision to see being spa as a great way to meet its goals, as will its professionals, and will welcome the challenges it brings.

WHAT'S IN IT FOR ME?

A professional in a spa concept salon will have high-quality specialty and customer service training to bring her up to the spa level. However, she must *want* this training, seek it out, and be dedicated to carrying it to clients in her care. She must see it as a personal advantage to her or she will not be successful. Following are some of the advantages of achieving spa concept to the professional. As a result of a dedication to spa concept training:

1. The professional becomes a spa professional—she is no longer a manicurist, pedicurist, or nail tech. A spa professional has achieved the highest level of expertise in each area of her specialty and in spa concept skills.

2. A spa professional feels a new respect from the clients and her coworkers. She will no longer be doing manicures and artificial nails; she will be doing spa treatments, spa manicures and pedicures, and possibly artificial enhancements, all at a higher level of expertise that others will note and respect.

3. A spa professional will feel a new confidence in her work and her judgements because of supportive new knowledge and her higher expertise, developed through exceptional training and over time during the treatments.

4. The spa professional has a *career* not a job. Her feelings about herself, her work, her position, and her place of work reflect this change in attitude.

5. The spa professional feels and portrays an inclusion in the overall goals of the salon, her colleagues and her clients. She knows that her success is directly tied to the meeting of her goals and those of her colleagues and the overall spa.

6. This spa professional works in a nail spa, not in a nail room or nail salon.

7. The successful spa professional is making more money because she is doing her best to meet the needs of her clients.

"Real" Spas

Many successful day spas and their professionals have attempted to meet this challenge of reaching spa concept in their nail department, and many have succeeded. However, in too many, exit surveys reflect that clients do not find the nail services to be special enough, memorable enough, and professional enough in the nail department. Owners are frustrated by the results of these surveys and the attitude problems they must handle in their nail departments.

Spa and salon owners are verbal about their problems in their nail rooms. During a conversation with one spa owner he waved his arm at his nail department, and said, "If I could, I'd board it up!" Why did he feel that way? Because:

> The department wasn't "paying its way" in the spa.
>
> The technicians were difficult to work with.

The nail department had the highest rate of absenteeism among the professionals.

The nail technicians were unhappy and always complaining.

Their client care was mediocre, sometimes poor, rarely superlative, according to surveys.

His complaint is common to owners of large salons and spas concerning their nail departments. What could be a root cause for the unsatisfactory performances and attitudes of these technicians? After all, many are working in the finest salons and day spa in their areas, yet they are performing poorly and complaining constantly. Could it be routine for manicurists to complain and be poor performers?

I have found one common denominator that will predestine this unfortunate situation. That common factor is the *training* policies in the salon or spa, specifically, who gets it and who does not get it. What about the quality of training? Retraining? It is interesting to compare the nail department's training with that of the training provided in their other departments. This is how it usually goes in many of the salons and spas that have "problem nail departments:"

- The hair department in every good salon or spa is of high quality. The salon's quality of service in this department is perpetuated by a strong apprenticeship program that is led by a well-trained educator. The apprentices sign on expecting an extended time of advanced theory and are provided abundant hands-on and technical training. They are trained, tested, and mentored to great length before gaining their chair.

- The skin care departments require extensive training time, formal classes, and mentoring that will ensure the quality of the service. Departmental trainers obtain advanced training repeatedly and the product companies are expected to support the professionals with extensive classes. The training can take months before the professional is allowed to work on a client alone or get her "room." Retraining is extensive and constant to maintain consistency in expertise and introduce new services.

These departments are provided the educational tools for supporting the new professionals as they develop into the kind of employees the salon wants. Re-education to maintain these skills is a continuing project. As a result, most of the professionals in these departments can be expected to reward their owner with excellent work and attitudes.

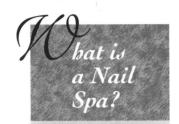

What is a Nail Spa?

Nail salons and nail departments, whether in a salon or spa, must meet all the following challenges to be considered a nail spa:

The Menu

Services are offered in a balanced, well-planned menu.

The services meet the needs of the clients.

Enough time is allotted for the services to prevent hurried activity and stress for the professional and the client.

Costs of the services and charges for them are carefully defined to allow profitability while not charging above the market.

Services are supported by fully skilled professionals and appropriate space and equipment.

The Environment

The nail spa has a healthy, nurturing ambiance, from the waiting room throughout.

The comfort and convenience of the client are the primary considerations.

The manicurist must be clean and neat at her work station.

Sanitation and clean technique are important and taken seriously.

Pleasant sights and activities only are observed by the client during her service.

The overall environment must be comfortable and relaxing.

continued

The typical attitudes of owners toward their nail departments, however, was expressed by one owner: "How difficult can it be to do nails?" or, "How much training do they need *just to do nails*?" The technicians are provided a weak training program when hired, then occasional updates are offered by manufacturer's reps, at best. The departmental trainer is not given special training or provided support materials; she "just knows how to do nails." She passes her expertise on to new personnel, who are seated at a table within a week or two and perhaps given written sheets as references as to how the manicures and pedicures are done. They struggle to gain speed, suffering humiliation when the clients are unhappy with having an obvious novice. They are, however, readily reprimanded each time a client complains—with the resulting dollars taken from their pay—and are told to straighten up their act—after all, anyone of the hair designers could sit right down and do nails. How hard can it be to do a good manicure? As a result, the nail professionals feel insecure about their performance, have no consistency of services, and develop more poor habits and bad attitudes.

The clients see poor professionalism and service and complain in their exit surveys. Then, the owners of these salons and spas malign their nail departments and wish they would disappear. "What can I do about the nail department?" they say, with frustration.

These management attitudes toward nail departments permeate the spa industry in varying degrees of severity. They are reflected in the spa industry's general attitude toward manicuring. For instance, in the definition of day spas by day spa industry, nail care is *optional* in a spa, which can be seen as meaning it is unimportant, or extra. However, the clients must not agree with this definition because they usually insist on manicures when they go to a spa. (Conversely, many do not request a hair service.) For that reason, most spas provide manicure services, though some reluctantly, reflecting an "and manicures, too," attitude.

Such owner attitudes result in confirmation of the owner's resentful attitude: the work in the nail room is poor, the technicians are sullen or prima donnas, turnover is high, and profits, if any, are low. Some owners just give up and get rid of the department because it was problematic, a description used by an owner of a well-known spa toward his former nail department, which no longer exists.

The reality is that manicuring is as much a part of spa concept as facial and body skin care. How can a spa visit be complete if the client's face and body are treated, but not her hands? Beauty goes clear to the fingertips, and well-trained spa manicure professionals are the ones to do the care.

Wise real spa owners will train their nail professionals in the spa concept and provide them with the necessary skill training, environment, equipment, and supplies to accomplish it. They will define their expectations carefully and consistently follow through with the retraining support to maintain this spa concept at the highest level.

As a reward for their efforts, the owners will see the nail *spa* become a profitable and pleasant *spa concept* area within an integrated organization. It will become an important contributor to the organizational goals; the nail technicians will become "spa professionals in the nail spa," not "nail techs in a nail room," and will reflect the attitudes of professionals who respect their clients and the workplace, not those of complaining prima donnas. No longer will the technicians feel like outsiders who are maligned by the other professionals and the management team. Best of all, they will gain the respect of their clients. The client surveys will put them at the tip of their list, not the bottom!

Analysis-Driven Manicures

Successful nail spas follow the same service philosophies in their nail services as successful spa skin care departments, that is, each service begins with an analysis of the client's skin, then recommendations are made for the particular service to follow. These services are *analysis driven*, not menu driven. The analysis by the nail professional at the beginning of the service is the pivot from which the remainder of the service springs, as it does in skin care. It points to the procedures that will fulfill the service needs of the client's skin as well as the nails, plus the recommendations for the client's home care needs and future appointments.

In the purest form of spa concept, the client does not 'appoint for' a particular service in an analysis driven service. Instead, the client will come in for an appointment; then, after analysis of her hands and nails, the professional recommends the appropriate service(s) that will produce immediate improvement in her skin and nails. These services are chosen by the professional for their specific nurturing and rejuvenating skin care and their techniques and products that will meet the needs of the client's skin and nails as she has seen them during the analysis. The client who is accustomed to spa concept defers to her professional's expertise and the service proceeds.

During the analysis and throughout the appointment, the client is educated toward extending and nurturing the improvements achieved by the service through home care products and future nail spa care. Ultimate results are described, future care is recommended, and the client is instructed in the procedures for and the importance of home care.

The Service

The manicurist is analytical and knowledgeable.

The manicurist is friendly, open, and oriented to the clients.

The manicurist gives her full attention to the client.

Client analysis is performed before every service.

Service recommendations are provided, with full explanations.

The client's skin is included in the service on an equal basis with nail care.

The client's care is the primary focus of the conversation.

The service is pleasant and complete.

The products are appropriate for the services and produce the results desired.

The Skills

The manicurist is highly skilled in both skin care and nail services.

The manicurist can answer questions forthrightly, or will find someone who can.

The manicurist has a firm and confident touch.

Purposeful repetitive steps within the skills are used.

Consistency is seen as important to the maintenance of service quality.

The Home Care

Home care products are recommended and considered an important service to the client.

Home care products are in the salon and ready for the client to purchase.

Home care products target the specific needs of the client as seen in the analysis.

continued

The manicurist has full knowledge of the ingredients and uses of the home care products.

The manicurist fully trains the client in his or her part of the partnership in care.

The Nail Service Closure

The nail bed is prepared for the retention of the polish.

The client leaves with a perfect polish application every time.

A drying procedure is routine.

Reappointment is always suggested.

A specific service is recommended for her next visit.

Home care products are packaged for the client.

Home care routine is explained fully.

The Follow-up

Thank you cards or calls are made to new clients to ensure satisfaction.

Personal marketing techniques are routine.

Service surveys are used and monitored.

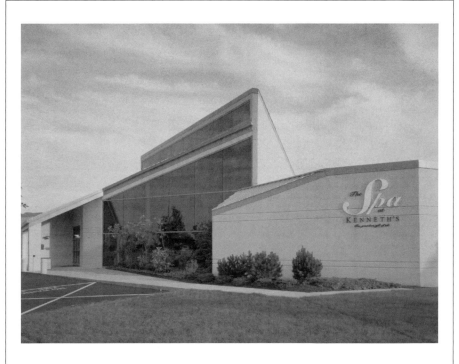

Why We Upgraded to Spa Manicuring

Kenneth's Hair Designgroup is a number of upscale and highly respected hair design salons in Columbus, Ohio. Ken Anders, owner, closed down several salons in an upscale side of the city in 1996 and combined them into a large and beautiful salon (above). A year later he added a day spa—a client walks through glass doors and enters a beautiful and relaxing day spa to receive wonderful treatments from highly skilled spa professionals who use the highest quality products and treatments available. The salon and day spa is 18,000 square feet of elegance.

Kenneth's Hair Designgroup and Day Spa had a beautiful manicure department, connected to a relaxing and elegant nail spa next to it in the day spa. His people were trained in some spa treatments, but he felt there was something missing. Anders' statement follows:

"We pride ourselves in offering the highest quality services available, using the best products available, then we charge accordingly. We felt we hadn't done that to the degree our clients are accustomed to in the nail department. For that reason, we decided to upgrade to spa manicuring.

continued

"The upgrade was done with a concentrated training, one day at a time, with the professionals learning the last step prior to adding each new one. It encompassed the basics of skin care and consultation on through to new custom manicures and pedicures, home care product training, and new spa products that were chosen specially for our salon.

"The technicians were ready for this upgrade and were excited, as well as the management team and the other professionals in the day spa. It took time, since we chose to start again at the basics, but the results have been beyond what we'd imagined. The income of each individual professional is up, their confidence and pride are up, and home care sales are up beyond any possible expectations. The clients love the new services and have responded with eagerness, so the income of the nail spa is higher than it has ever been. Best of all, however, is the improved outlook provided the nail spa professionals, and their wonderful and professional demeanor. They're a highly-contributing part of the spa now, right up there with the estheticians!"

The clients in analysis-driven services respond in a positive way that is familiar to skin care professionals. They respond to the professionalism that is reflected and the results that are achieved; manicures and hand treatments become an important aspect of reaching goals for healthy and beautiful skin and nails.

Over time, most clients will come to see the spa concept as an important aspect of their beauty regimen. However, in some nail spas, analysis-driven manicure appointments cannot be accomplished in its purest form because the clients will not accept making appointments that do not have a designated service assigned. Some never will. These clients will continue to 'appoint' for the services of their choice, and the spa manicurists will continue to work within that routine. However, this should not discourage the professional from performing analysis—a service name on the appointment book is not written in stone. During the analysis, she recommends a particular treatment manicure or treatment and teaches and recommends home care.

The concept, ultimately, is the same except that the technician at times may be making recommendations for *future* appointments, not current ones, if there is not enough time reserved for the recommended treatment. For instance, at the first appointment, possibly the client is on the book for a 'manicure' that has the minimum time reserved. During this appointment, the technician can recommend a spa manicure (which takes the same amount of time) and prepare the client for future analysis-driven appointments by practicing analysis and making service recommendations. For a client with dry skin, she can say, "Your skin needs more intense moisturizing and hydration, so we need to book 45 minutes for your next appointment for a hydrating manicure. You will like the softening and moisturizing results."

Be certain to inform her of the higher cost, such as, "The hydrating manicure is a great healer and moisturizing treatment and is $X more." If the client appears to be hesitant with the cost upgrade, offer the upgrade for the price of the first manicure as an introduction to the service, allowing her to see the difference during that appointment. Then, the receptionist places "hydrating manicure" on the book, allowing the appropriate time.

Each time a client comes in, her card is pulled (or her computer file is recalled) to inform the manicurist of the client's condition at the last appointment and the defined needs that were seen then. After the client is seated, the manicurist reaches for her hands and analyzes her service needs. (Fig. 1–7) Soon the client will expect an analysis whenever she comes in; she will put her hands out and say, "What do you think?"

Analysis-driven manicuring requires the spa manicurists to know what to look for and what to do to correct what she sees (see Chapter 2). It requires *responsible* and *analytical* decision-making on the part of the manicurist, and then prescriptive recommendations toward meeting the goals she has discerned the client wants to meet, today, tomorrow, next week, and next month. It requires a skillful and caring trained professional who can affect these results for her client, right before her eyes…that takes training.

Upgrading to Spa

The steps to becoming a nail spa may require several changes throughout the nail salons and departments. It can mean changes in decor toward a more subtle environment. It may mean changing the music and straightening and removing clutter in the area. It may mean some serious control of fumes. It probably will mean further training for the professionals and a search for appropriate products and some equipment. It certainly means a new view of manicuring.

This new orientation may require a difficult change in the professional orientation of some nail spa manicurists, such as from "I already know how to do manicures," or "I hate manicures. No way," to "I want to

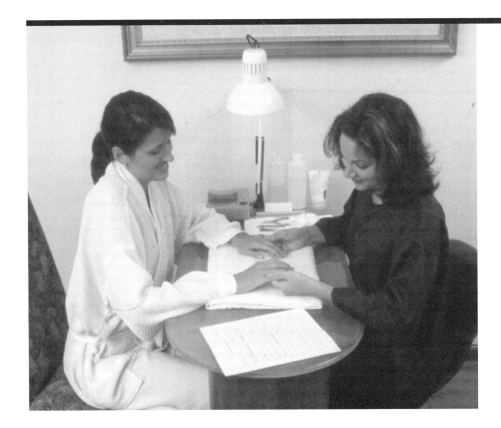

Figure 1-6

A preservice analysis
is performed on the
client's hands.

meet all my client's needs," and "I want our area to meet spa parameters, just like the rest of the spa (or salon)." Learning skin care and hand treatments and changing the outlook and procedures toward spa concept will require setting skill goals and training. Structured training and skill measurements should be implemented and reimplemented.

PRINCIPLES OF SPA CONCEPT SERVICE

Spa concept training moves a nail department to a new orientation:

> From service focus to recommendation orientation
>
> From salon and professional focus to client orientation
>
> From nail care focus to skin and nail health and beauty

To do so, certain service principles are targeted to meet the concept of spa. These service principles can be seen by the professionals as:

- *The focus in a nail spa is the client and her care, not the employees or getting the appointments done.* This focus should be present in every interaction the professionals and auxiliary personnel have with the clients. The entrance routine, menu, ambiance, services and treatments, home care products—all are focused on the client's needs, not toward fitting them conveniently into the salon or technician's overall day.

- *Nail spa professionals are alert for, observe, and act on details.* Nail spa professionals conscientiously maintain the small details as closely as the larger ones. (Details are important to spa clients and are mentioned in the surveys.) The nail spa environment is clean, quiet, and friendly; the supplies are neat and there to use. There are no hassles, just a focus on providing more than the best service for this client. A nail spa moves beyond the clients' expectations. Nail spa services must bring "aaaaahs," even during the maintenance services.

- *Nail spa professionals are highly trained in spa specialty skills.* Nail spa professionals are trained in specialty skin care and spa skills appropriate to meet their client's needs in addition to enhancement and manicure skills. Their services always begin with an analysis. Their manicures, treatments, and enhancements are always a step above those of other salons in quality. Their appointments always end with recommendations for home care maintenance and future service.

- *The nail spa professional is results oriented.* This professional can look at the client's skin and nails and recognize what will meet the client's needs both today and in the future. She can envision how the hands, nails, and skin will look after appropriate treatments as home care. She can convey to the client the services and home care that will result in her hands and nails becoming what she wants them to be. If that is impossible, she will inform her as to what can be done to make her situation more tolerable, with appropriate maintenance appointments and home care.

- *The nail spa ambiance is quietly rejuvenating.* Successful nail spas and their professionals know that recharging and recuperation are not done to the tune of *intense* music, blaring bass treble in the background, and the heavy odor of acrylic fumes. The environment is relaxing and pleasantly aromatic because the professionals know a tense client is not in the healing mode...or a good mood. Spa clients want to enjoy where they are and respond to the nurturing of the manicurists through the quiet and healing aura of the environment.

- *The owner and managers achieve and maintain spa concept as an overarching philosophy of service.* The overall environment in any organization stems from the focus and example of those in charge. If management does not work diligently to achieve and maintain spa concept and actively support the service principles among all the employees, both auxiliary and professionals, spa concept will not exist for long in that nail spa…or in an overall salon or spa. Success comes from defined expectations and a superior training program.

SPA CONCEPT AS A DECISION-MAKING TOOL

Spa professionals and managers who understand spa concept soon begin to use it as a decision making tool. When decorating is to be done, when client care is being defined, or even when an activity is considered in the presence of a client, the question will become "Is this spa concept?" or "Is this appropriate for a spa?" A spa concept manicurist will look around her work area between each client and consider "What will my client see when she sits at my table? Does everything in her sight appear as it should in spa concept?" A professional designing new services will consider "Is this service going to be spa concept?" An owner designing a new menu will wonder "Is this menu a 'salon menu' or a 'spa concept menu'?" The spa concept becomes a professional standard to achieve and maintain in all aspects of the business.

Comparing salon standards to spa concept standards for the purpose of using them as decision making tools is simple: just look toward the results to be achieved. In a salon, the result focuses on a 'look,' an image, an appearance, something that is immediate and the result of the art of the professional. In spa concept that is true also, but there is more. This result is produced in a calming, rejuvenating, and regenerating atmosphere, producing something for the client that is *inside* her as well as on her exterior. It will be longer lasting, possibly even a *building* treatment that looks toward a later, more correcting and healing result.

Seeing the differences between the two is important to understanding the use of the spa concept as a decision making tool. Every aspect of the professional life in a spa concept salon, spa, or nail spa should be measured against this standard. If so, the clients will see it as what it should be — a place to go for relaxation and rejuvenation as well as a beautiful look — because it is really "spa."

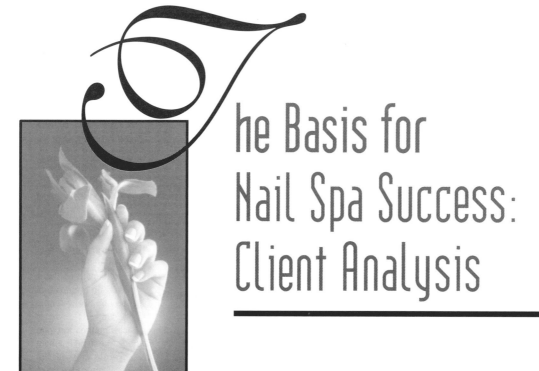

The Basis for Nail Spa Success: Client Analysis

2

OBJECTIVES

At the end of this chapter, you should be able to:

- Perform a formal analysis of a client.
- Recommend the appropriate treatment for the client.
- Classify the skin types relevant to the hands.
- Name and identify skin care conditions of the hands.
- Recommend skin care treatments for hands of the client with artificial nails.
- Analyze the nail plates of your clients.
- Name the six conditions of natural nail plates, plus normal nails.
- Determine the condition of each client's nail plate.
- List the professional products and equipment for performing a service on natural nails.
- Discuss formaldehyde in nail polish and strengtheners.
- Define a regimen for the improvement of natural nails.
- Educate the client on the precautions and use of nail strengtheners.
- Define the nail plate conditions on which formaldehyde nail strengtheners should not be used.

Hair designers are taught in beauty school to do a consultation on each client. Skin care professionals are taught a detailed procedure for skin analysis as the pivotal point of their service. It has been proven that professionals who follow this training stringently produce better results and are more successful in their careers than those who do not.

Manicurists are not routinely taught detailed analysis or consultation. As a result, clients call for an appointment in a salon and the service is placed on the book as the client defines it. "I want to make an appointment for a manicure," she says; that is written in the book and that is exactly what she gets. She comes in, receives the basic or hot oil manicure she requested, and she leaves, with nice polish and a pleasant service, but not one that was specifically designed for her needs, through analysis. No questions are asked by the manicurist, and none are expected by the client. After all, this is "just a manicure."

Now, however, clients are demanding more than the mechanical no-improvement manicures of the past. They want effective and lasting manicures that will fulfill their personal needs and desires, along with treatments that will aid them in correcting the conditions that make them feel their hands are "old and ugly." To accomplish this, manicurists must become more involved than before in the needs of their clients. An analysis of the condition of the client's skin and nails including her questions about her personal goals and needs is the first step, just like the hair designers and estheticians do at the beginning of their services.

What is the difference between analysis and consultation? *Analysis* determines what the condition of the nails and skin is through observation and questions. *Consultation* determines the service that will be done through suggestion. Analysis is the mechanical aspect of determining the needs, whereas the consultation suggests the specific services or programs. For the purposes of this book, we will call this entire step "analysis."

Most of us do some form of analysis. At a minimum, we look at the appointment book to see what the client has scheduled. Then look at her hands to see how much time she is going to take. Then we start. Our analysis is mostly for *our strategic purposes*, not for meeting the client's needs. Too bad—both of us are being cheated.

The *spa professional* performs an actual client analysis. She looks closely at the client's skin and asks the appropriate questions. She:

1. Determines her client's service needs

2. Assesses her home care needs

3. Provides her with information about how, what, why, and when for her future appointment needs

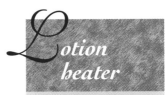

Lotion heater

The heater that was used in the traditional hot oil manicure is not in favor in spa manicuring, as it only heats or treats the tips of the fingers when it is used as intended. However, one can be used to add a dimension of luxury to the manicures. Heat a single treatment of the lotion chosen for the manicure in the plastic tray, then dip the lotion out of it with a spatula when it is needed.

Many salons give the lotion a "push" toward the right temperature by placing the tray in a microwave for 3 to 5 seconds first, then just placing it in the heater. (It takes too long to heat otherwise.) The heater set on low will maintain the warmth nicely. For sanitary reasons, only one serving of lotion should be in the paper liner at a time. The liner is thrown away after the service, along with the tiny amount of remaining lotion.

4. Recommends the appropriate home care products and briefly describes their use

5. Suggests and performs the services

As a result, the professional receives an enviable monetary reward for meeting the client's needs and improving her skin and nails.

No spa services or skin care can be done properly without a formal analysis—the foundation of the spa concept. It is the primary factor that sets the spa manicure professional apart from the traditional and full-service manicurist. She is set apart even from the upscale manicurist, who may be analyzing the needs of the client's nails, but not including her skin in the analysis.

FORMAL ANALYSIS

A spa professional does a formal analysis when the client sits down, after the entrance routine, and before any service is begun. It is a *separate part of her service.* This is how it proceeds for a new client:

- The new client sits down, the spa manicurist suggests she place her keys and any other items in a routine place at the table, then is made comfortable. The manicurist knows what she is scheduled for (No, not, "So. What are we doing today?"), has clean table towels down, and polish removal supplies ready. Nothing else is on the table top. (Fig. 2–1)

- The professional discusses the client's general health, using the spa questionnaire she completed as a resource. The repeat client is briefly questioned, asking if there are any

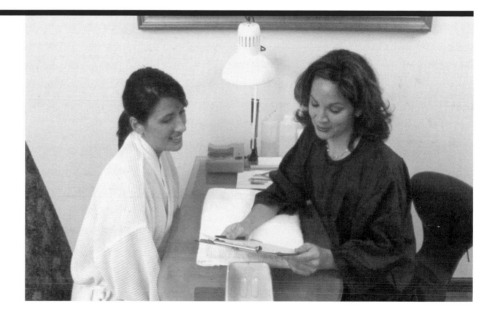

Figure 2-1

The manicurist reviews the completed questionnaire with the client.

changes in her health. The professional will usually know of the regular client's health changes from conversations, but must take care to be certain she is aware of any others.

- The spa manicurist removes the polish, keeping her attention on the client's hands and nails. She looks up and asks, "What would you particularly like me to do for your hands today?" or, "At their best, how would you like your hands and nails to look when you leave today?"

- The professional then gets her ready for the analysis. She says something like, "Let's take a look at your hands and nails." (Fig. 2–2) She takes the client's hands, one in each of hers, and places them, palm down on the table towel. She touches the back of one hand, and picks it up to look at the knuckles. (Fig. 2–3) She looks at each finger to check out the cuticles, touching them.(Fig. 2–4) She turns the hand over and touches the palms and fingers. During all of this, she is telling the client what she is seeing. The hand is placed back on the towel and she goes to the other hand and does the same thing.

- Now, she proceeds to the skin on the arms and elbows. (Fig. 2–5) "What can we do for these areas today?"

- Next, the professional considers the condition of the client's nails. The client with natural nails will receive a different analysis than the client with enhancements.

- The manicurist discusses everything she sees with the client and asks questions that will focus on the conditions of her

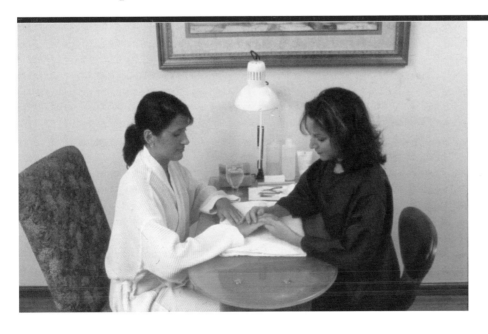

Figure 2-2

The professional begins the examination of the client's hands.

Figure 2-3

Every aspect of the hand is examined, including the skin and the nails.

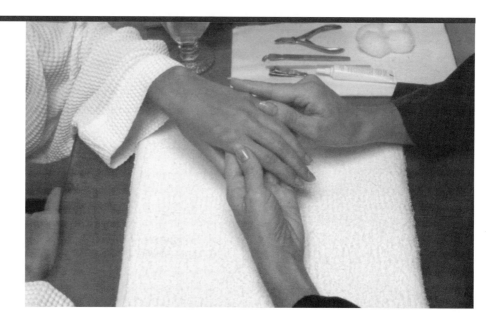

Figure 2-4

The professional explains what she sees as she examines the hand and nails.

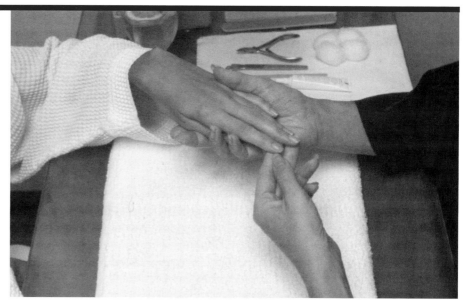

skin and nails and on her lifestyle. Examples of questions for a new client would be, "Are you in a lot of water frequently?" "Is your facial skin dry?" "What do you do at work?" and "What do you do as a hobby?" Regular clients will get a slightly different analysis than a new client because the professional is familiar with her skin and nails, and usually with her lifestyle. (She wrote notes on her card or in her computer file when the client was first treated.)

- Finally, the spa manicurist recommends the treatment(s) for the current appointment, both for the nails and skin, suggests the needed home care, and mentions possibilities for future appointment needs.

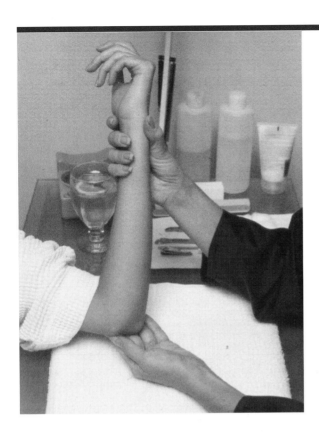

Figure 2-5

The professional analyzes
the arm and elbow.

"Ready, Set, Go"

Analysis is the signal that the manicurist is prepared to provide a service and will recommend which one it will be, according to the client's needs at that time. New clients like this routine and are always amazed at the professionalism of it, if it is correctly performed. Regular clients will know and expect the manicurist to do it at the beginning of *every* appointment. These trained clients treat their manicurist as the expert as early as the second appointment. It is rewarding for both the client and spa professional.

The secret? Analysis must be done consistently in the *same way, every time*. This is not the only correct routine; there may be another that will better fit your needs. The important thing is that one is adopted, that it is made an integral part of your table routine. It is the same at every appointment.

The spa professional will immediately notice the new respect she receives from her clients. **Important:** In your routine, *touching* the area you are analyzing is important. The client will follow the touch with her eyes, become more involved in the process, and even add to your analysis by voicing concerns she wants considered.

New clients will respect and accept this routine immediately, more than your regular clients who were accustomed to the old "sit-and-talk-about-their-life" routine. They are used to the "no commercial

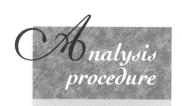
During analysis the spa manicurist will:

- Determine the condition of the hands and nails.

- Establish the probable causes for any problems.

- Suggest the appropriate service regimen for the appointment.

- Prescribe home care products and usage.

- Suggest changes in client activities that may be contributing to the problems.

- Outline a specific program for improving the look and condition of the client's hands.

stuff" relationship (no matter that their hand and nail conditions did not improve) and to initiating their own treatment. Therefore, a spa manicurist may have to implement her new professional analysis more slowly into the routine of her regulars. This may mean just mentioning what is seen, with a few recommendations, in the beginning. Do not fail to do it, though, and be thorough in the chosen explanations. It is important to your client's welfare…and to the professional's. The regulars *must* be upgraded to spa as quickly as possible because they are the basis of the professional's and the salon's income.

Keep in mind that regular clients tend to note what other newer clients are getting; they will be more open to the new routine if they see it being done by every professional on other clients in the nail spa. If their hands and nails are not analyzed, some will pout and say, "Why aren't *I* getting that done to me?" So, do not be too quick to deny a regular client the formal analysis; she may respond very well to your new philosophy. Always be obvious with the analysis movements and observations, so other clients can see what is being done.

Preparing for a Successful Analysis

The manicurist must be able to gain the client's trust and cooperation for the analysis to be successful, and client must believe in the recommended services and programs. Her respect for the spa manicurists professionalism is the key to gaining this cooperation. For that reason, professionals must be educated thoroughly on the skin and nail problems that they will be facing *before* undertaking even the first formal analysis. If they are not knowledgeable about all the possibilities, the client will sense hesitation (or worse, read it as 'salesmanship'), and the situation may become a disaster. To be blunt, if professionals are not ready to do their homework and skill, forget analysis…and forget spa manicuring. Professionals who try it without the proper training are perceived as unknowledgeable and unskilled, and their service results will be the same as before the attempted change, or worse. The client may even become irritated at the suggestion and leave the client list.

After becoming familiar with the symptoms and causes of each condition and where they fit into your service recommendations, the nail spa is ready to design the new menu of services and implement the overall change (see Chapter 15.) This is not a quick change, a call-the-distributor-and-add-the service thing. It takes time, planning, and investigation by a patient and focused manager who has the goal well defined. For a large nail spa, it may take months; for even a salon with only one nail professional, it will take thought, time, and practice, which can take weeks. The most important preparation the professional can do is to understand the various skin conditions and how they look and feel. This learning process takes study, practice, and observation of as many hands as possible.

SKIN CARE AT THE NAIL TABLE

Expectations for our services are different from those for the face or body. Clients are educated and accustomed to patiently awaiting results for a month, or even 3 to 6 months for changes in the face and body. "It takes time to remove wrinkles," they are told about their faces. "One pound a week is the safest way," they are told about dieting. They even willingly accept "no pain, no gain" as part of getting into shape, as well as months of time and effort.

We have, however, spoiled them in the nail salons. "New nails in one hour for a new perfect life!" They walk in with terrible looking nails, and walk out with great-looking ones. We have to live up to this reputation. To be successful in a nail spa, the hand, arm, and elbow skin care must be "Ah-ha!" services. We have to show quick and lasting results or clients quickly get discouraged and disappear.

Classification of Skin Types Relevant to the Hands

To fully meet the expectations of our clients, we must be knowledgeable about the skin and how to deal with its problems. Usually this will include "skin typing" so that we can know how to make decisions regarding procedures and care.

Skin types for the face are listed as normal, dry, oily, combination, acneic, sensitive, mature, and dehydrated. The types for the hands are basically the same, although no oily or acneic skin will be seen. Following are a list of the usual types, as they are seen on the hands.

- *Normal*—Normal skin has a healthy glow and smoothness, with wonderful elasticity and moistness.

- *Dry*—Dry skin will be resistant to movement across its surface, feel coarse and tight, and appearing dull in color.

- *Dehydrated*—This skin will have fine lines and wrinkles and will appear thin and stressed.

- *Sensitive*—These hands will react to many products, may appear irritated, and will probably have a dry, possibly even rough surface.

- *Mature*—These hands will be creepy in appearance (usually dehydrated), with wrinkles. Hyper-pigmentation may occur in varying degrees, according to the amount of exposure to sun over the years.

- *Environmentally exposed*—These hands may be one or more of the above, due to overexposure to chemicals, water/solvents, the sun, the wind or weather, and possibly abrasion. Callusing is often present on these hands.

A spa manicurist will be proficient at determining the skin type of her clients, through a thorough analysis, and know immediately what she will recommend for treatments, future appointments, and home care.

SKIN CONDITIONS OF THE HANDS

What is first? The skin care type or the skin condition? The skin type will usually develop particular conditions under certain influences, that is, dry skin will become chafed and rough if exposed to cold environment and not treated with the necessary lipids. The following are descriptions of the most common skin care problems seen at the nail table.

- *Chafed and dry*—This client's hands are dry and scaly; they may even crack open over the knuckles and become sore to the touch. The client with such hands may constantly have her hands in water as a part of her work or home routine, or she may be required to wear gloves constantly in her work and she does not wear glove liners. She could be a dental hygienist, a homemaker, or a bartender. She may be constantly exposed to harsh weather conditions, or she may just have naturally dry skin that gets much worse during winter cold and wind. She is ashamed of the appearance of her hands. They are painful and sometimes ruin sheer clothing when rough tags catch on delicate fibers.

- *Dry skin with extreme roughness along the sides of the fingers or thumbs*—This client may have either environmentally dry skin or systemically dry skin (usually it is environmental exposure to harsh conditions). Whatever the cause, the condition is exacerbated by calluses. Some of her calluses may be roughened, causing the surface to have areas that may be described as 'mini-cuts' that do not fully penetrate the callous. These cuts may collect dirt or dyes that discolor the mini-cuts. This client may have given up on her hands. They look and feel like alligator skin, tear and run clothing, and attract negative comments from anyone who touches her hands.

- *Rough, torn cuticles* — This client's hands may or may not be dry. If they are, they will vary in their degree of dryness. (I have seen clients with this condition with only minimal dryness on their hands, overall, whereas other hands can look like leather or are chaffed.) The program will include manicures for the hands, with an addition of treatments for her cuticles. Her cuticles are dry, rough, and torn for many reasons. The cause may be using of paper or other "oil-sucking" materials in her work; or she may be a nail or cuticle biter who tears her cuticles chronically or a person who must wear gloves all day in her work and is not wearing glove liners. Whatever the cause, she is often in pain with infected and torn cuticles, and is always concerned about the way her hands look.

- *Dry, leathery skin* — This client's dryness causes her skin to appear hardened and almost smooth or leathery. Many of her cuticles are callused along the sides of the nails, from behind the stress points to beyond the free edge. Her cuticles and hands tear her clothing and elicit thoughts in those that touch them similar to the ad on TV where the alligator walks by the camera. This client is extremely embarrassed and will do *anything* her spa professional suggests that will help curtail the condition. (She has already tried all the drug store and department store remedies.)

  Her condition can appear to be systemic, meaning "it just is." She has a dry body, overall. The deep-rooted cause is not for us to question or diagnose, but it can be caused by illness, genetics, drinking and smoking, anorexia, among others. An environmental cause can be excessive sun exposure. Right along with her leathery hands and skin, this client may have obvious and severe wrinkles on her face unless she has invested much money and time toward improving them.

- *Aging, wrinkles and loss of tone* — This client has severely wrinkled and dry hands. The cause can be genetic, aging, and possibly overexposure to the sun. Her elbows will be severely wrinkled also. Only a plastic surgeon can take tucks to remove all the wrinkles, but regular manicures and treatments can make obvious improvements that these clients will see as miracles.

- *Micro-pigmentation problems, such as "age spots."* — The tendency toward pigmentation changes is usually genetic, but can be triggered by sun exposure and hormonal imbalances. The problems can be improved dramatically by skin treatments, but cannot be totally corrected except through heavy duty peels by the plastic surgeon. Manicures can bring dramatic improvements, however, for the client who commits to the suggested program and sticks to it.

- *Sensitive and/or allergic skin (chronic symptoms)* — This client's skin is sensitive and sometimes sore. Chaffing can occur with any weather change or any irritation at home or work. The causes can only be determined by a dermatologist. Our job is to help her toward comfort, without causing additional irritation of any kind.

- *Normal skin with seasonal and environmental dryness* — This client usually has healthy skin, but may experience dryness caused by seasonal changes or some change in her activities. Our job is to help her through these changes and back to "normal" through systematic analysis and recommendations for treatments and home care. Any dryness really annoys these clients.

- *Elderly skin* — These clients have thin skin that is easily torn and bruised. Special care must be taken to prevent damage to them.

- *Overgrown cuticles* — These clients have cuticles and pterygium that have grown excessively onto the nail plate and are tightly sealed to the nail plate. They are embarrassed about the condition of their hands, but have tried everything to control the growth to no avail. They will welcome weekly prescriptive manicures if the professional can aid them in attaining the appearance of normal. This process will be slow, but it can be accomplished. The condition will return if clients cease manicures and the attending home care.

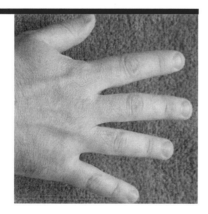

Figure 2-6

A chronic nail biter.

- *Nail biter* — These clients can be any of the above, but with the added complication of chronic nail or cuticle biting. These are special clients who need encouragement and patience, though firmness. (Fig. 2–6.) When they come to a professional, they are ready to quit, but they need help from a professional; the spa manicurist. This is a program that may or may not show immediate results, but will, with time, include alternative 'busy hands' recommendations, nail care and skin care treatments, and support from the manicurist. These clients will never leave you when they reach their goal!

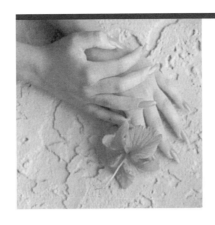

Figure 2-7

A client with artificial nails is interested in hearing about skin care treatments.

- *Client with artificial nails* — The addition of professional skin care treatments to the regimen of the client with artificial nails should be easy because, she already appreciates nice nails. She will be interested in nice skin. (Fig. 2–7.) The analysis will usually prove that the client's skin falls into one of the above conditions. The skin care services are usually greatly appreciated by these clients, although the initial services may have to be free introductory offerings.

A New Niche: Natural Nails

When the new manicure trend began a few years ago, it struck fear in the hearts of us, the nail technicians. We were afraid acrylic nails were going to disappear. But that has not happened. Instead, it appears to be a response of a whole new niche of clients, clients who would never have appreciated artificial nails. Our clientele has embraced a new group of clients who before would never have come into our salons. Then, these clients expanded their demands to skin care and here we are, at spa manicuring, a new level of service for us.

To meet the demands of these clients we must be able to meet the needs for their skin and their natural nails. To do so, we must include their nails in the analysis step of each service.

NAIL PLATE ANALYSIS FOR CLIENTS WITH NATURAL NAILS

Analysis is not complete without a thorough look at the client's nail plates and recommendations for their care and improvement. Clients define the appearance of their hands by the health and beauty of their nails.

Fingernails are important in our society. We are judged by their appearance and condition, including acceptance or rejection for relationships and positions of employment. Their appearance may affect

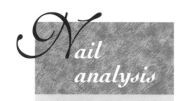

Nail analysis

A complete nail analysis is an important aspect of the client's visit to a spa manicurist.

our self-esteem, our posture, even our facial expressions and body positioning. Nail technicians often see dramatic improvements in posture and facial expressions, solely because of a positive change in the client's fingernails.

The condition of their fingernails is what brings the majority of clients into nail salons. Their nails are a "mess," and they want us to correct that condition, *immediately*. However, until recently most of us knew little about improving the appearance of the natural nail plate so we just applied enhancements and considered the problem solved. Few of us knew methods for quickly and dramatically changing natural nails. With the new products and treatments we can now recommend, we can feel confident the client's nail plates *can* show immediate improvement and their nails can become beautiful natural enhancements to their overall appearance within a short period.

The secret to successful retention of these new clients is offering them services that obviously and quickly show results. To do this, a spa manicurist must *look and listen* during analysis in the first moments of the service. One of the steps is defining the condition of the client's nail plates. The spa manicurist picks up the fingers, touches the nail plates and the cuticles, and tells the client what she sees. She then recommends professional services, home care products, and treatments to improve the nails and discusses reasonable expectations for their improvement.

The analysis routine is the decision of the spa manicurist, but an analytical look at the nail plate should not be seen as an afterthought or separate procedure. The analysis of the skin and nail plates should be one procedure. For example, while the spa professional is looking at the skin of the fingers, she can perform the nail analysis and make appropriate recommendations. Or, she can complete the skin analysis and recommendations, then slide to the fingertips, note the condition of the nails, and make recommendations for their treatment.

Nails change with the seasons, lifestyle changes, health issues, stress, and any number of other influences, so nail plate analysis should be performed during every appointment with the same necessary stop-look-listen focus as with skin analysis. When changes occur, the manicurist notes it within the steps of the analysis and enlists the client's cooperation toward making adjustments in her treatment and home care recommendations.

CONDITIONS OF THE NAILS

A nail professional should first learn the detailed anatomy of a nail and the nail bed for the nail plate analysis (see Figs. 2–8 and 2–9). Then, she must learn *conditions of the nail plates* and treatments and manicures that will improve them. These conditions are of the *nail plate surface*; they are not diseases or disorders, such as *onychorrhexes* or *onycholysis*, though they may also be present. Nail conditions may reflect a deficiency, however, such as dryness or peeling, as a result of such diseases or disorders. (Diseases and disorders should be referred to a dermatologist and not diagnosed or treated by a spa professional.)

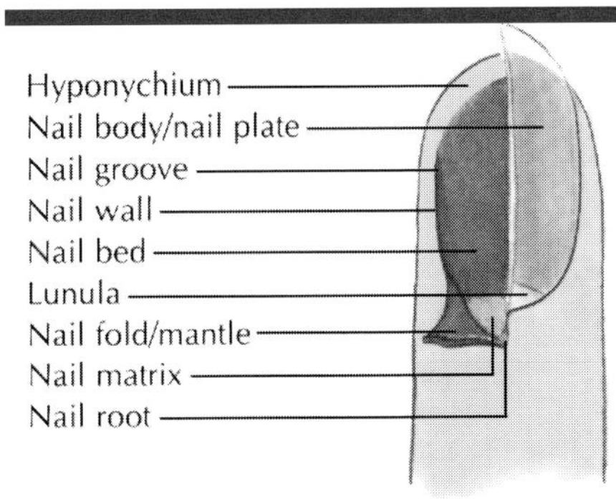

When the spa professional is defining the condition of a client's nail plate, she will usually see one of seven conditions, each with its own causes and treatments. Normal nails are a maintenance procedure, however, not resolution of a nail condition. These conditions are:

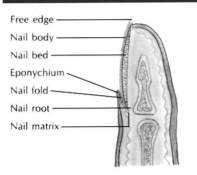

Hyponychium
Nail body/nail plate
Nail groove
Nail wall
Nail bed
Lunula
Nail fold/mantle
Nail matrix
Nail root

Figure 2-8

The nail and its many layers.

Free edge
Nail body
Nail bed
Eponychium
Nail fold
Nail root
Nail matrix

Figure 2-9

Side view of the nail layers.

- *Normal nails* — These nails are strong but flexible with an apparent free edge that is shaped and beautiful. They resist breakage and have a uniform and healthy coloring in the nail bed area and a uniform and whitened opacity on the free edge.

- *Peeling/layering nails* — These are the problem nails that we most commonly see on our clients. The nails lose the natural adhesive that bonds the layers of the nail plate then peel apart, layer by layer, until they are thin and weak. Next they tear and there is no free edge.

- *Brittle nails* — These nails seem strong, then the free edge breaks with very little pressure. There is no crack, the nail just comes off in a chunk. Clients may refer to the break as a 'snap,' describing the suddenness and possibly the sound.

- *Eggshell nails* — These nails are thin and weak, bending easily. The entire free edge will peel off with very little pressure. They bend and straighten with little effort. Many times they appear to 'lay' over the end of the finger, having no arch of their own. (Fig. 2–10)

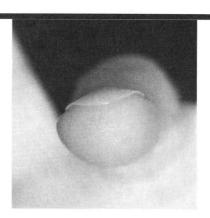
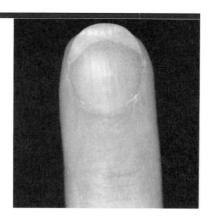

Figure 2-10

Very thin and weak nails are called *eggshell nails*.

- *Lacy nails* — These nails are weak and floppy also but may have some areas on the free edge that seem to be thinner than the rest, giving them the appearance of lace. Some areas will appear clear, others will be opaque, causing the lace like appearance. They tear easily and have rough snags that tear clothing and hosiery. (Actually, clients with lacy nails seldom have a free edge.) These nails are truly an annoyance to the client because they seldom can grow to any length.

- *Stress breaks* — These nails appear to be *too strong*. They will be strong and appear thick and healthy, then suddenly there is a deep break at the stress area of the nail plate in the side well. A frequent cause is long-term overexposure to high percentage formaldehyde resins in some nail hardeners. (Fig. 2–11)

- *Enhancement nails* — These nails will vary in health according to the skill and care of the application technician performing the enhancement procedure or according to the health of the client and her nails, and according to the general health of the client. Over-prepping and etching will cause thin nails and curved markings in the nail as it grows out. Incorrect use of a nail finisher during finish of the acrylics will also cause severe trauma and curved markings in the nail plate. Correct application of products will not produce an unhealthy nail, though it may be more flexible for a short time after removal of the enhancement product.

Figure 2-11

Overly strong nail causes a *stress break* in the nail plate.

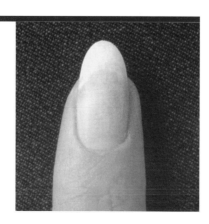

Treatment Possibilities

After determining the condition of the nail plate, the manicurist decides what treatment is appropriate and informs the client. Such choices were limited until recently when manufacturers began recognizing the potential of natural nail care and developing new and effective products to enable us to meet the needs of the new niche of clients. Manicurists who wish to take advantage of this market should develop a repertoire of both professional and retail products, solid information concerning the products, and analytical skills for their effective recommendation. They should then develop appropriate routines for the use of the professional treatments and home care products at their table.

The nail professional's professional products for enhancing the natural nail plate include:

- Natural nail emeries—these emeries are 240 grit and higher, and will not initiate layering on the free edge.

- Cuticle oils and treatments—these products enhance the condition of the cuticles and stimulate and moisturize the natural nail.

- Nail strengtheners and treatments—nail conditions will improve with the proper treatment product and regimen.

- Buffers—gentle buffers shine and smooth the nail plate.

A prerequisite for success in natural nail treatments is intricate knowledge of the professional and home care products. A spa manicurist must study the treatment ingredients within the professional and home care products and know how each will affect the clients (see Chapter 11.) Classes, beauty industry books, and articles in the trade magazines can empower the manicurist to suggest safe and highly effective treatment plans for their clients. This knowledge, coupled with consistent analysis procedures for changing the recommendations as indicated, will perpetuate the beautiful results that clients desire.

NAIL PLATE TREATMENTS

Recommendations of nail plate treatments can be complicated. Many are in multiple steps and will produce great results on certain nail plate conditions. However, their use is not as simple as it seems because, used incorrectly, they can cause problems. Many will produce a great improvement initially, as intended, but a change must be made to a different product (or "step") to maintain that improvement. The responsible nail professional will know her products well and alter the recommendations, as needed.

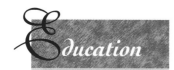

Natural nail conditions are a challenge requiring appropriate education, a discerning eye, and proper decision-making. For instance, products for brittle nails are the opposite end of the spectrum as products for peeling nails, so the recommendations and treatments must be different. Normal nails need only be "maintained" and protected. Products that harden the nails should not be recommended for normal nails because the nails may eventually become too hard and dry. They may become brittle and begin to snap and break.

Formaldehyde Nail Hardeners

The use of formaldehyde nail hardeners is a controversial and polarizing subject. However, a book on natural nails must address it to be complete, so I will reluctantly proceed. (I may be hearing from those on both sides of the controversy.)

Individuals who are exposed to high concentrations of formaldehyde can develop sensitivity and allergic reactions if they have such a propensity. Products at the highest allowable concentration (3%) may cause allergic reactions in such individuals even with short-term use, causing an itchy rash on the skin surrounding the nail plate and increased pigmentation of variable brown beneath the nail plate. Even a slight indication of these symptoms requires the client to cease using the formaldehyde-containing product. These symptoms can progress to leukonychia and onycholysis.

Products of lower concentrations of formaldehyde are reasonably safe for temporary use, but the responsible manicurist must remain constantly alert to any comments or symptoms that might indicate a potential allergy. Let me emphasize again: even the slightest itching indicates a possible manifestation of allergy and product usage should cease, immediately.

For years, polish contained a small amount of formaldehyde and produced a low percentage of allergic reactions. Then, though the percentage and possibilities were very low, it was removed from most polish products. Now, most polishes contain no formaldehyde, but strengtheners do, and they are the best-selling treatments on our shelves.

Many manicurists and their clients are unnecessarily addicted to the use of these products because they show immediate results. The chemical hardens the nail by chemically cross-linking the nail proteins and most clients experience positive changes in the cosmetic appearance of their nails with no allergic reactions. Clients who never had a free edge can grow beautiful and strong nails. However, I have learned from many years of experience with clients with natural nails, that the hardness developed with formaldehyde is not truly a stronger nail; it is a rigidity, a stiffness, due to the cross-linking, which means it may begin breaking easily with long-term use of the products as the nail becomes brittle.

Now, I am not discounting the responsible use of these products. I believe there are safe ways to use them for most clients and have recommended them to my clients for years. However, a knowledgeable and responsible manicurist will not put them on at the highest concentration and continue use indefinitely. She will use analysis at each appointment, moving to a lesser product concentration as the client's nails become beautiful, then suggest a step down to an even lower concentration. Finally, the client's nails are so improved she can use a non-formaldehyde product, one she will use indefinitely to maintain the health of her nails.

An example of this treatment plan is the one I use for layering and peeling nails. These clients may have nails with a long-standing condition, or it may have started recently, possibly from a change in activities, stress, or illness. Whatever the cause, there has never been an indication that this is a disease or disorder treatable by medications or ointments. To the contrary, no medications have improved the condition, even treatments that later cured the systemic diseases that may have contributed to the peeling problem. It seems to be perpetual—once the nail is dry and the interlayer adhesive is gone, layering or peeling continues. Any minor trauma further loosens a layer toward the posterior of the free edge and the layering continues until it is specifically addressed with a treatment that successfully stops the peeling.

Over the years I tried diligently to solve this problem. I glued the free edges, I peeled then glued, I oiled, I tried everything that was sold; nothing seemed to work except covering them up with enhancements to hide them. Then the higher percentage formaldehyde resin products, in steps, appeared on the market. The clients loved the results and so did I. My clientele with natural nails grew quickly because they told their friends, who told their friends that I had the "magic touch."

Then I noted some problems. The clients would get "stuck" on the high-level formaldehyde product I recommended at the time. They were addicted! Then 6 months to a year later, their nails would begin to snap. "What is happening here," they would ask. "What have you done during these manicures to cause this?" They were horrified, and of course, it could not be their "miracle" product, it had to be me.

Finally, I realized that even though I know about the side effects of formaldehyde use from my dental background, I had not transferred that information to nails. Formaldehyde is drying and a stiffener, *I had*

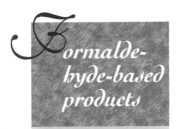

Formaldehyde-based products

Use a step-wise treatment regimen when using products with a formaldehyde base.

to insist they change to products with lesser levels of formaldehyde as their nails improved or the nails would eventually begin breaking. (The newer product lines recommend this in their information; the product I recommended initially was vague on this issue.)

The routine I have found to be effective involves the use of one of the higher percentage formaldehyde products initially, but *only for a short time*. The amount of time I have found to be best for the client is the time required for growth of new free edge from the hyponicium to a reasonable length. (This may be shorter time of use than the client desires, of course.) For most of my clients this is about the time it takes to use the first half ounce bottle or, at most, two of them, or from 6 weeks to 3 months. Then those who have severe peeling are stepped down to a lesser amount of formaldehyde for one bottle, then to the lowest for one bottle. After that, I routinely take the clients off the formaldehyde products completely and recommend a bottle of good non-formaldehyde nail conditioner. This is used *forever* as a protectant and barrier in their nail's own natural moisture.

Clients with only moderate or minor peeling should use the higher percentage products a shorter period of time, proceeding to lower percentage products faster and using each concentration for less time. I often have them use the formaldehyde product for the time of one bottle *or less*, then take them immediately to a non-formaldehyde product. Or, I recommend the second highest level of formaldehyde, next the lowest, then on to the non-formaldehyde-based products. These clients should be switched to a non-formaldehyde conditioner as quickly as possible.

The clients should be informed of the precautions necessary in the use of these products. They should be informed of the potentials for allergic reactions and dryness and taught to monitor their nails, in tandem with their manicurist. They should be taught how to apply the product safely—away from the cuticles and not on the skin—told of the potential drying effects, and the need for "stepping" to different products as the condition improves. Most of all, they should be informed that they are an important partner in the improvement of their nails: if they do not do their part, their nails will not improve. That responsibility includes returning routinely to the nail spa for their manicures.

The product should be sold as a treatment program, a means to their goal, beautiful nails, and not as a maintenance product. The program should be fully monitored to alleviate the possibility of producing an "addict" client, one who will decide that the *product* is the reason for her beautiful nails, not the care and recommendations of the spa manicurist. The uninformed and addicted client may change to another salon and manicurist to try to retain the formaldehyde product in her manicure regimen.

The potential for the peeling of the treatment product from the nail plate in the early treatment phase should be explained to the client. It may peel off in sheets during the first week or two of the product's use before establishing effective cross-links in the surface of the nail plate. I explain the peeling as an indication that the product is working—"just take it off and start over when/if the peeling occurs. It will stop when the cross-linking is established." If left unexplained, the client may become disgruntled. "This isn't working," she may say, and ignore the professional's recommendations for her hand care. She will stop the treatment and stop coming in for manicures.

These clients must be taught proper home care to support these products or their nail condition will *never* completely disappear. They should be told when and how to use the product, reminded to use gloves when using solvents, and instructed in all other precautions for damaging nails. Cuticle oils should be included in the home care for improving the health of the cuticles. The client must be brought into the regimen as a partner toward reaching the goals for it to work.

Spa manicurists must routinely analyze their clients' nails for possible changes. Adjustments in health, weather, and lifestyle will cause changes that may require modifications in home care products, even a shift to a stronger strengthener temporarily.

The Nonformaldehyde Conditioners

Clients with some conditions should *not* use formaldehyde products. Clients with brittle nails, normal nails, or stress breaks should use a good non-formaldehyde product from the initiation of their care. Normal nails will be dried out by formaldehyde products and will become too rigid. Brittle and stress break nails are already too dry and rigid; formaldehyde products would only worsen the breaking. These nails will respond well to the non-formaldehyde nail conditioners, the function of which is to hold in the nail's natural moisture and promote flexibility and health, not harden. These nails also need daily application of good essential oils, with cuticle and matrix massage to stimulate the natural oils and nutrients in the skin and the matrix.

Brittle and stress-cracking nails will take time to correct—until the formaldehyde-treated nail plates grow off (if that is the cause), and the new, stimulated and more flexible nails grow out. In the mean time, a spa manicurist can manage the breaks with natural nail repairs, proper nail shaping, and length management. Clients respond well to this management of the conditions and consider their nails "healed" long before they are, usually.

The perfect nail conditioner has not yet been found, but nail companies are working toward it. Personally, I expect several on the market soon, as a result of the intensive research into potential chemistries. When it does—it may be happening during this writing—and I hear about it, I will test the validity of its claims at the table; if it proves to be that perfect nail conditioner, I will be the first to tout its discovery. Why would any manicurist choose to continue to use a chemistry that has potential for allergic reactions and backlash damage to the nails if one is available that does not? If you know of one already, let me know! I want it!

The manicurist who searches for classes and information on treating natural nail conditions, and uses them at her table, will develop pride in her manicure skills that may be equal to or exceed her pride in her enhancement services. When a client tells her that she loves her long, beautiful natural nails, then adds, proudly, "and they're *mine*," she experiences a professional pride she has never felt before. The client will send "her spa manicurist" all her friends who have natural nails.

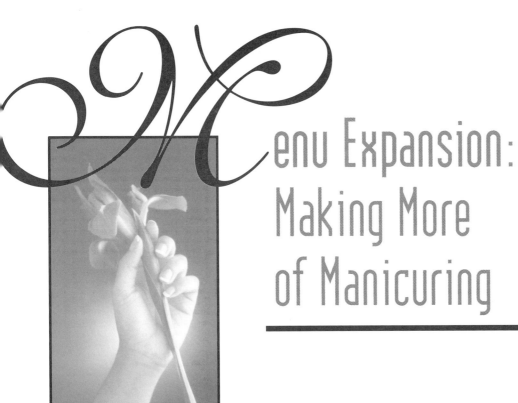

enu Expansion: Making More of Manicuring

3

OBJECTIVES

At the end of this chapter, you should be able to:

- Evaluate the nail spa menu for needed changes.
- Define treatments, manicures, and programs.
- Determine fair fees for the basic manicure.
- Use mathematical analysis to determine whether manicures are profitable.
- Add skin care treatments for clients with nail enhancements.
- Use double station technique for adding skin care.

A client's dissatisfaction eventually shows up in the lack of profits of the salon. The upscale salon nail department may be sluggish or never quite paying its way. Growth in a specialty nail salon may be stagnant or the clientele decreasing, causing the salon to not be as profitable as it could be, or it may struggling just to stay alive. In a spa, the nail room may be the lowest profit area overall and be consistently on the bottom of the client exit surveys. The owners of these businesses become frustrated, and the technicians sense it; both will agree these nail departments need rejuvenation.

What can be done to solve this dilemma? More training? Different technicians? More technicians? Redecorate? Some of this may be true, but before management begins to make such changes they need to evaluate the service menu. They need to start with revitalizing and restructuring the menu. Several questions should be asked:

1. *Are the services too traditional?* A menu that focuses on the traditional manicure, even with an added traditional paraffin treatment, does not provide the lasting results that clients require for today's stressed skin and abused nails.

2. *Are the services memorable?* Manicures must be more than a maintenance appointment or clean-up job. Clients now are requiring 'aaaahs!' in their manicures that rejuvenate them and restore relaxing balance to their hectic lives.

3. *Are the services providing immediate improvements in the client's skin and nails?* Improvements to the skin and nails must be directly attributed to the manicures or treatments that are done in the nail spa if the clients are to return consistently.

If the service menu still contains only the 'good old' basics,' it is not surprising that the manicurists are not at the top of the client service surveys or that clients are not returning with enthusiasm. They are not receiving quality services, and they know it by looking at their hands. Why bother? They have many other places to spend their money.

THE SOLUTION

Salons must have the edge against the salon across the street. A specialty nail salon must be the best in its niche. An upscale salon must perform services that will set it apart and produce good reasons for clients to return regularly. A spa nail room must provide ambiance, overall atmosphere, and spa level services. The wisest move toward achieving this differentiation in the nail areas would be to become a *Nail Spa* and that means a nail menu that offers spa-level services.

Developing a new spa concept menu requires, first, an understanding of the philosophy of spa concept, the benefits of upgrading the specific spa manicures, and then acquiring the skills essential to achieving these memorable results. This new menu must reflect the new spa abilities of the manicurists. It should no longer have the word "basic" on it; new manicures, treatments, and programs will be listed, with their description and benefits.

THE NAIL SPA MENU

A nail spa menu will offer a description of the needs of a salon's clientele. The only limitations the menu will have are these needs, the limits of the chosen product line(s), current development of treatments, and the expertise of the professionals. (Fig. 3–1)

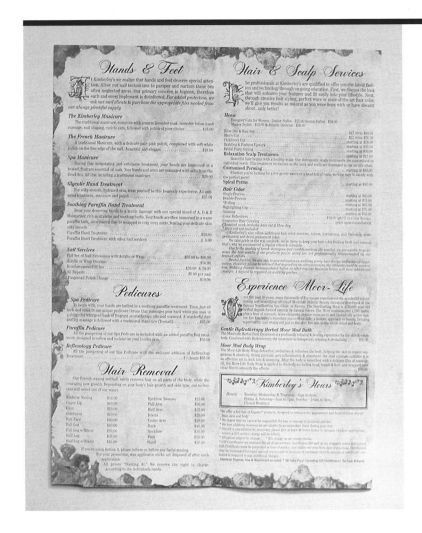

Figure 3-1

The nail spa menu offers a description of the salon's services.

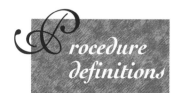

- *Treatments* are separate activities that show a dramatic difference for the client, as designated by their name. They can be performed as a separate service or as part of a manicure procedure.

- *Spa Manicures* are services with defined procedures and use high-quality professional products. They include work on the nail plates and contain massages, cuticle work, and polish renewal. They may or may not contain treatments. The names should tell the story of their expected results.

- *Programs* combine manicures and treatments in multiple services toward meeting a particular goal.

Within these limitations, certain criteria must be met in choosing the services. Each service must:

- Reflect an immediate improvement
- Provide the client the opportunity for attaining her goals
- Sound wonderful, using words that evoke relaxation and pampering
- Sound memorable and rejuvenating

This is spa. However, it is more than just adding a few spa specialty services and attaching the word 'spa' to the salon name. This menu reflects the attitude, ambiance and activities philosophy of spa concept. It suggests that skin care will be integrated with nail care and that the client will feel wonderful during and after the service. All this must be reflected in the design and content of the menu.

The overall physical design of a spa-type menu reflects subtlety and, again, the feelings the client will experience while in the salon. The colors are not bright and the print bold and demanding. The pictures are muted and show persons relaxing and obviously enjoying revitalization and rejuvenation. The information is in spa language. The menu supports what the client wants in her spa experience and assures her that she will get it if she comes to the salon. She will have a spa concept experience.

The menu should be interesting in a nail spa and may be quite long. It contains spa-type manicures, treatments, and programs; manicures are different from treatments, and a program is an expanded combination of the two. It may even include 'packages,' purchases of multiple predetermined services (see Chapter 14).

Following is a brief description of the manicures, treatments, and programs that will be presented later in this book. Nail spas may include them all, different ones, or only a few, according to the needs of their clientele. Many nail spas will include a basic five, and train their spa professionals to suggest the others according to a client's needs (upgrades). All these finite decisions are the final decision of the menu designer. The following are only suggested as possibilities for a nail spa, not as a final and defined menu for a nail spa.

The (name of the nail spa) Manicure. This manicure is a salon's basic manicure service but with an added dramatic twist or, a new, realigned procedure. It will give your clients immediate and more lasting results for maintaining the health and appearance of the skin of their entire hands and their nails. Best of all, this manicure sets the basic manicure above those of other salons. (In this book it will be called the 'new basic.') It is designed for clients with normal skin.

The Spa Manicure. This manicure is the above manicure including the arms and elbows plus placing the hands in plastic wrap or thin, long baggies after the massage, then wrapping them in towels. The hands are wrapped in a towel or placed in terry mitts. The name spa requires that the client be sitting in a quiet, calm atmosphere, allowing her relaxation and rejuvenation, and the use of high-quality lotions and oils that produce great results in the procedures. (Fig. 3–2)

The spa manicure produces immediate results for the client's skin. The wrapping and warmth produced by the plastic encourages the natural moisturizers of the lower layers of the skin (dermis) to come into the closer surface layers of the skin (epidermis). Further, the nutrients and moisturizers of the treatment lotion will be more readily absorbed into the warmed, open 'pores' of the skin.

The effects on the plastic-wrapped hands define the name for this manicure as 'spa manicure' because it produces the spa effect, holding the client's natural heat and moisture. For that reason, many nail spas choose this as their most basic service manicure; they believe that the spa effect is necessary to meet the spa concept philosophy. The charge is appropriate, of course. This manicure is the foundation for most of the treatment manicures in spa concept.

Terry mitts can be heated slightly in the microwave or warmed towels can be wrapped around the hands and arms outside the plastic. Avoid

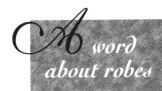

A word about robes

Clients who receive services in virtually all day spas are generally provided robes to wear. While this is an example of another touch that can give a spa "feeling" to your salon, it is not necessary. Many clients may feel more comfortable wearing their street clothes, rather than changing to a robe, and many salons and nail spas do not offer them as a part of their ambiance.

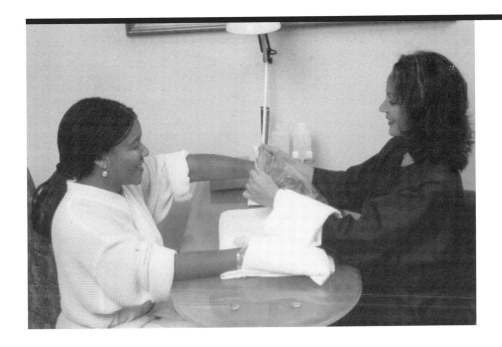

Figure 3-2

The quiet and calming atmosphere provides complete relaxation.

choosing the use of the electric mitts in this service because they make it too similar to the hydrating manicure, possibly removing it as a menu possibility. (This would be a mistake because the hydrating manicure should be seen as an important upgrade from the spa manicure.) The electric mitt treatment in the hydrating manicure is longer and more involved, yes, but the similarity is still too apparent.

Hydrating Manicure. The spa manicure is the base service. After the hand is massaged, treated, hydrated with the appropriate lotion, and placed in the plastic wrap or bag, it is placed in electric thermal mitts during the time the other hand is being treated, plus a 'set' time. (Fig. 3–3)

Before you say, 'What's so new about that? I've been doing that manicure for years,' read the procedure chapter. It shows two important additions to the manicure make up the differences and provide the ability for an immediate improvement in the skin.

Aromatherapy Manicure. This manicure is a 45- to 60-minute hydrating manicure (above) that further incorporates aromatherapy oils throughout the service. These same aromatic essential oils are used in the massage to invigorate and relax the client, are in the cuticle oil, are possibly infused into treatment towels, and used as a compress during the service; the rejuvenating treatment perks up the client's skin. The clients *love* this manicure and will become addicted to the relaxation and rejuvenation it provides them while it is treating their skin to hydration and nourishment. The manicurist must be familiar with essential oils to do this manicure prescriptively.

Figure 3-3

The hydrating manicure, and use of electrical mitts and lotion improve skin almost immediately.

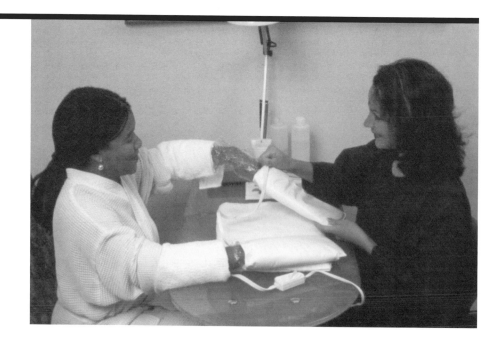

Herbal Hand Treatment or Manicure. Exfoliating herbs can be used as a prep, a treatment, or part of a structured manicure. Exfoliating herbs, which have both physical and chemical exfoliating abilities, are the working element of the treatment or manicure. The herbs produce immediate re-texturizing of the skin surface and remove surface roughness. These herbs have a wonderful side benefit that will be discussed chapter 5.

Emergency Care Treatment. This treatment is for the client who has sore and chapped hands. It is a hydrating and healing treatment, with soothers and healing lotions applied, under mild heat for immediate relief of the pain of chapped and raw skin. This client must do intense home care, and possibly return for two to three treatments the first and possible the second week, then weekly until her hands are normal.

Paraffin Treatment. This treatment can be recommended for treating systemically dry skin, for comforting arthritic joints, or even as a relief to winter 'blahs.' It can be used alone as a 'stop in for a dip' or as an element of a treatment manicure. In the stand-alone service, the hands, arms, and elbows are cleansed, prepped, and treated generously with the appropriate lotion. Then the paraffin is applied to seal in the lotions and enhance their effects. The treatment is removed after 10 to 15 minutes. The treatment lotions and oils for use under the paraffin are determined during the analysis. This treatment is a superior enhancer to other treatments.

Sloughing. This treatment or manicure is a physical exfoliation that *mechanically* removes dry, scaly skin and the discomfort that accompanies it. It can be a preservice treatment to manicures (an add-on), a named manicure on the menu, or a treatment service in itself. For example, the treatment can be an addition to the hydrating manicure and listed as a sloughing manicure on the menu, or it can be a separate sloughing treatment. As a treatment, it involves the skin and cuticles of the client, not the nails, with no nail shaping or polish application. (A treatment can be two to three visits the first week, with the manicure only occurring once in that time.) The products for sloughing can be lotions with rough granules or salt glow products, among many.

Sloughing, however it is offered, is for the client who wants immediate relief from roughness caused by systemically, environmentally, or occupationally dry skin. It is highly appreciated by those who need it and produces dramatic results. Many of the treatment manicures will involve a preparation of the skin with a sloughing treatment. This prep step prepares the skin to accept the treatment oils and lotions.

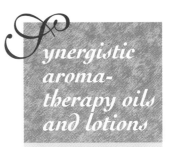

Synergistic aroma-therapy oils and lotions

Many nail spas chose synergistic lotions, oils, aromasols, and pedicure soaks that can be used throughout a manicure or pedicure. They have identical aromas and are used in each of their functions within the service. The clients relax into the subtle aromas, and they can purchase retail products from the line to use at home. For instance, the professionals at Kenneth's Designgroup and Day Spas, Hilliard, Ohio, allow their clients to choose the aroma they wish to enjoy, then the service products are each of this aroma. The massage oil, the lotion, the aromasols for use of the towels, and the pedicure soak all are a synergy of the wonderful aroma she chose. The experience is pleasantly aromatic and relaxing, just what the client ordered!

Exfoliating. This treatment or manicure is for those who have very dry but probably not rough skin on their hands (leathery). Clients with systemically dry or sun-damaged skin are candidates, as well as those whose chapped skin has healed. Clients also respond to its anti-aging qualities and abilities to even coloration of the skin. They must commit to weekly manicures/treatments with their eye on the future result. The treatment encourages the exfoliation of the old and damaged outer layers of the epidermis, revealing younger, softer skin. This service and the retail products that go with it are expensive, and involve a chemical exfoliation system of AHA (alpha hydroxy acid) and/or BHA (beta hydroxy acid) products. (For our purposes, sloughing is mechanical, exfoliation is chemical.) The exfoliating treatment will be a 15- to 20-minute procedure.

The treatment is skin care and has nothing to do with the client's nails. The professional interested in doing this service is a careful professional with expertise in skin care. Clients love the results and see an overall improvement in the skin on their hands.

The cost of the treatment will be according to the area exfoliated, that is, if the hands alone are exfoliated, the cost is less than if the hands and arms or the hands and elbows are included. Prices should be set carefully, according to the amount of time and chemicals used for the treatment.

Hand Facial. This skin and cuticle treatment can be done as a separate appointment or as a preservice to a manicure. A 'hand facial' is a procedure similar to the facial routine in which the skin is deep cleansed, exfoliated and then a treatment mask is applied. The purpose is to deeply cleanse and hydrate the skin and cuticles, often it is done as an alternate appointment to the sloughing manicure or the exfoliating manicure, or it can just be a treat to those who may be sick of the winter or effects of the sun on their skin.

Age-Defying Treatment. This skin treatment will take years off the texture and appearance of the client's hands. It produces excellent results over a period of time on the discolorations of age, with quicker results on the texture and appearance of the skin and cuticles. The clients must commit to weekly manicures and/or treatments (a program) with their eye on the future result. The program involves AHA skin treatments, hydrating masks or treatments, and home care products, including a hydro-quinone treatment if the client has age spots. It can be a listed manicure or a treatment separate from the client's nail service, as with the exfoliating treatment or manicure.

A manicurist who is interested in seeing overall improvement in a client will be interested in performing this service. The client's hands will look younger, take on a more even and youthful glow, and appear more toned. Those who commit to this service love the results. The service and the retail involved are expensive.

Treatments and Treatment Manicures. Treatments using various products from the salon's facial line, or a line chosen for this particular purpose, will provide results the clients will love. For instance, a manicure can be developed using the vitamin C serum from the product line that will brighten and tone; an algae mask will deep cleanse and tone. The trick is to do the manicure similar to the facial routine with minor logistic adjustments, so the product will reach its treatment potential.

An innovative manicurist knowledgeable in skin care can develop interesting manicures for her department. The aid of an esthetician who understands the differences in skin structure and environmental exposures on the hands can be helpful.

These manicures are becoming an interesting focus in nail spas. Consumer beauty magazines are mentioning that clients are seeking out dramatic hand treatments to produce the results they are enjoying on their faces and body. Products are available that can enable us to produce those results if we develop the procedures.

Acrylic Manicure. This manicure is for acrylic wearers, performed between fill appointments, or before their fill. Client analysis determines the actual treatments needed for the skin. In the separate acrylic manicure, no work is actually done on the acrylics unless a repair is absolutely necessary, but the rest of the manicure is the same as the prescriptive treatment or manicure. (The enhancements are just 'there.') It treats the client to the skin care and pampering that clients with natural nails enjoy and improves the condition of their skin to a point of added satisfaction. (Fig. 3–4)

Some salons have an acrylic manicure on their menu for smoothing, shaping, and repairing the client's acrylics between fills. It has nothing to do with the client's skin. Another name may be designed for the treatment manicure or it can be booked simply as the spa manicure or other prescriptive manicures. The menu designer will be the one to make this decision.

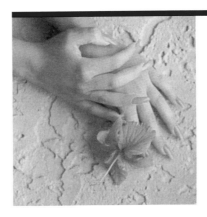

Figure 3-4

Clients that enjoy beautiful acrylic nails also want beautiful skin surrounding them.

Acrylic Brightening Treatment. This treatment will whiten and brighten the acrylics, not treat the client's skin. As a former dental hygienist, this one was easy for me to develop! The problem with this treatment is that the materials have a tendency to dry the fingertips, so it should be used only every 3 to 4 weeks, when absolutely necessary, or when the client requests it. Personally, I prefer doing it before a fill, if it is to be done, and I add a hydration treatment to repair the skin and cuticles.

Hand Reflexology Treatment. This special tension-relieving massage can be an excellent short service or can be added to other manicures as a treatment. Fifteen minutes to a half hour should be the appointed time, as a separate appointment, but the best application is, of course, within other manicures and treatments, such as the hand facial, hydrating manicure, and so on. Ten minutes per hand is optimal within a manicure.

Male Manicure. Professionals must learn those little nuances that men like in their manicures, such as buffing and special polish that is not shiny. Otherwise, their manicures and treatments are the same as those for women. Manicuring a man can be intimidating for an inexperienced professional, so practicing on several male friends or employees (who will appreciate the free service) should be an important segment of training a new spa manicurist. (Fig. 3–5)

Nail Biter Program. The manicures in this program give extra attention to the cuticles, the skin, the nails, *and the client*. A schedule of appointments (or program) is set up for the client, including retail and home care products and instructions. Clients can quit a habit and grow

Figure 3-5

Manicures on men can be slightly intimidating for inexperienced spa professionals.

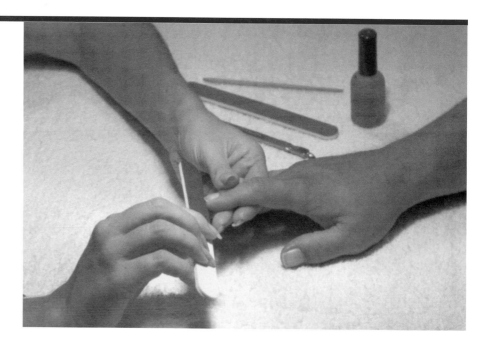

healthy nails with these manicures and the support of the manicurist. The specific manicures will vary, according to your analysis of the client's nails and skin at each visit. This client is a special person and must be treated in a special way. The program *works* and the clients become permanent residents on the manicurist's client list.

Nail Growth Program. This is a series of manicures or treatments for the hands, skin, and nails. It is a prescriptive program that aids the 'just-can't-grow-nails' client toward beautiful nails of the length she desires with the bonus of beautiful hands and skin. Each manicure is chosen according to the condition of the skin and cuticles, and each nail treatment is designed to bring the client's nails to good health. The program involves home care products, the matrix massage, weekly appointments, home treatments, and more.

The nail growth program is rewarding both financially and professionally for any professional who fully develops this clientele. The results are immediate and amazing. The clients see fast results and love it. They appreciate their manicurist, believe anything she says, buy anything she recommends, and send their friends in for services.

Acrylic Grow Off. This procedure is really a continuing program; the client is in it until the acrylics are gone. (A special number of manicures are not purchased, however. It is more of a goal for her weekly manicures.) It does include nail growth manicures, oils, and natural nail prescriptive products such as strengtheners and treatments for the skin. It is an alternative program to "soaking off" or other removal procedures and is an excellent retention procedure for a client who wants to remove the acrylics.

Clients will come from other salons to have their acrylics "grown off" when they hear about the manicurist's ability to gently grow off their acrylics, leaving healthy, strong, and beautiful nails. The procedure involves weekly visits for approximately 2 months, including retail. The client becomes a loyal manicure client. Further, this procedure can rid us of having to listen to the remark, "Those things ruined my nails!"

Manicures for the Elderly

This is not a separate manicure and will not be listed on a menu, but the subject deserves special mention. We have been taught about the care for their cuticles (no clipping); however, something more must be considered. *These clients have thin and weak skin on their hands, arms, and elbows, and their blood vessels have weakened walls.* Their skin will split with a carelessly firm massage, or an ugly bruise can develop right before your eyes. Massage these clients with the palm of your hand, gently and carefully, using mostly a 'rub,' not a massage. They love the atten-

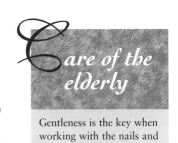

Care of the elderly

Gentleness is the key when working with the nails and skin of elderly clients.

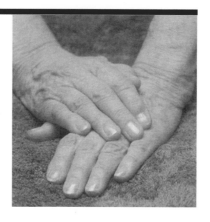

Figure 3-6

Clients who wish to change from acrylics to natural nails will appreciate a gentle grow off of the nails.

tion, but we must take care not to injure them or cause them pain or suffering. (Fig. 3–6)

Treatment of Arthritic Hands

This client is special and her massage takes special training. Her hands are stiff and painful—and will be even more so after the manicure if the professional does not use special care. She requires a gentle, slow-moving manicure, with special massage considerations, such as using only the palm of your hand to massage her and not the pressure pads of your fingers. This client's manicures are prescriptive but usually involve a paraffin treatment that offers soothing relief from her pain. Think of it as an 'aspirin' manicure. It will not cure her arthritis, but the welcome relief the client experiences with the paraffin will invite her to add the treatment to other manicures.

DESCRIBING MANICURES AND TREATMENTS IN SPA LANGUAGE

When a client peruses a *salon* menu, she probably will see the manicures listed in words such as 'The Basic Manicure' and 'The Hot Oil Manicure,' or 'Paraffin Manicure,' with little dots and the price. Some salons will put a description, such as, 'Includes a complete cleansing, filing, cuticle treatment, hand massage and polish,' followed by the dots and price. A few salons will be more elaborate, naming the basic with a more interesting name, such as the X Salon Manicure, with a description, such as 'Allow us to beautify your nails and skin with a shaping, cuticle treatment, a massage with a moisturizing lotion, and an application of a stunning color that accents your nails.'

In a nail spa, the menu is much more elaborate and uses an entirely new language to describe the services, including the manicures and treatments. In these menus, the *results* or the *skill* being performed are not the focus. A menu that is spa concept will focus on *feelings* and the *experience*, not the appearance or image of the outer results. Words such as *reawaken your senses…, experience the feeling of tranquility while…, feel rejuvenated after a…, relaxing in a luxurious…, while enjoying…,* and *pamper you while…* should be included in the descriptions. Service skills should be described with words that are used in spas, such as *Revitalize your skin in a…, Enhance the beauty of your hands by…,* or *A gentle exfoliation reveals vibrant and more youthful…,* and *Magical and softening essential oils will….*

These menus will allow the client to *see* herself experiencing the service in her own mind. She will see this as her 'time out' and will be ready to say 'aaah' as she is experiencing the service. The nail spa must, of course, be able to produce the environment and skills the description of the service suggests.

Designing a menu can be an agonizing experience (see Chapter 12.) One of the considerations should be cost. A nail spa menu will be more expensive because of the space that the service descriptions require. (The other spa services should also be described in spa language, except for the hair services. They still are focused on image and appearance.) The amount of elaboration should be balanced—too much sugar can make one feel sick, too little is bland and nonproductive. With a well-designed menu, the nail spa will note a correlation between the feelings it produces in the clients who read the descriptions and the increase in appointments for services. This is especially true for new clients and for current clients making appointments for the services they have never before experienced.

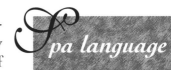

QUICKIE SERVICES

The title of this section is contradictory to spa concept but is a list of services that can be offered a client who is in for another service in another department in the salon. They can also be suggested as the manicurist or another professional recognizes an immediate need and minimal time is available. Some are add-ons, such as paraffin dips and toes-to-match, which are services that can be upgrades to other manicures and services.

Some 'quickies' can be looked at as clientele builders. Clients in other departments can be introduced to the nail spa through these services. Analysis should accompany the service to allow the manicurist to tell the client her further needs—and book her for a longer service.

- *Mini-manicure*—Some salons call this the express manicure. Polish is removed and the free edges of nails are smoothed a bit, but not reshaped. No massaging and no cuticle treatments are done. (If their cuticles are in poor shape, they need a full manicure. Do not be tempted to do this work in a mini-manicure or the client will never see the need to upgrade.) It should take no more than 20 minutes. (The relatively high cost, comparing the professional activity in it and the cost of the other manicures, is to allow the better manicures to seem a better value in comparison and to discourage a temptation to book the mini-manicure instead of treatments and full manicures.)

Many nail spas do not have this manicure on the menu, but it can be suggested as a service to a client already in the salon to introduce her to the manicure department. Other salons will keep it on the menu to get clients into the salon then will hope to introduce them to the more productive services.

- *Polish change* — This should cost the same as the mini-manicure and essentially be the same in activity. Clients who call to book a polish change should be offered the mini-manicure or a basic or spa manicure.

- *Matching toes* — When a manicure client wants her toes to match her fingernails but is between pedicures or cannot schedule one, book 15 minutes for this service. Charge an appropriate fee considering set-up time, and so on, if it is scheduled with and will fit conveniently inside another service such as a manicure. If it is scheduled as a separate service, charge the same as a manicure because set-up time and occupation of the pedicure room or area will be about the same as a manicure. (You should explain the reason for this to the client.)

- *Toe-nail shaping/polishing* — This service is for persons who are not able to shorten their own nails but cannot have pedicures, such as severe diabetics or hemophiliacs. Spray the feet very carefully, shorten/shape the toenails, and polish them; anything more is a pedicure. Charge a hefty fee; podiatrists charge them $30 to $65 for less — no polish and very minimal shaping.

- *Natural nail repairs* — Clients will especially appreciate their spa manicurist if their nail spa covers breakage 'emergencies' on natural nails as are offered for broken enhancements. The repairs can be resin or gel wraps, but the result must make the nail appear the same as the other natural nails; no bulk should be added.

For years I put acrylics on split natural nails as the repair but hated it. The nails appeared "fat" in comparison to the other nails, no matter how thin I made them. They snapped again in the same area, needing replacement, due to the thin application and weakness at the stress area where the break might be. They took too much maintenance and seemed to perpetuate the use of the acrylic on the nail due to rebreakage. The clients did not like it and neither did I.

The clients wanted a thinner application that resembled the shape of their other nail plates. Next, I tried gels, to no avail. They split even faster than the acrylics. Then, I tried fiberglass wraps. Fiberglass wraps held the break well without breakage due to the warp and woof of the fibers but seemed to fatigue and need redoing several times before stress breaks would grow out. Then, the warp and resin had to be placed back to the cuticle to maintain balance, causing a perpetuation of the wearing of the wrap.

Then I thought—How about trying a wrap with a gel over it? I tried this repair in 1990 and have been recommending it since then. I find it to be a one-application, grow-off repair that is strong, thin, and durable. The gel is flexible and absorbs trauma and seems to protect the fiberglass from fatigue while the fiber provides strength and flexibility. The repair grows off the nail without any need for refills and repairs if it is applied correctly. The clients love it because no observer can see the repair is there!

Some nail professionals use full coverage of the fiberglass wrap and gel. I prefer a stress strip, placing it across the nail at the break to absorb and equalize the trauma. Usually, I do not apply the gel clear to the cuticle and am careful to make the posterior area flat and neat. The enhancement will protect the nail until the break and the gel are grown off while the nail looks almost identical to the other nails.

- *Special occasion art*—Some nail spas can offer highly detailed and complicated nail art, others believe that nail art is not in the spa criteria. Some offer a short menu of specific artistic designs for special occasions. These beautiful 'quickies' should be designed to take only a few minutes and offered *specifically for special events and holidays*. The designs are regularly updated and only offered on a specially designed and updated list (no substitutions) as seasonal specialties. The clients have fun with them and the manicurists can, too. Charge a nice fee for them. (Fig. 3–7)

- *Waxing*—Hand and arm waxing services can be offered as add-ons to manicures for those pesky hairs on the fingers of some clients and for the clients who prefer hairless arms. The service is performed immediately before the manicure, though not before an exfoliation. (The sloughing step will also be canceled from the routine of those manicures on the

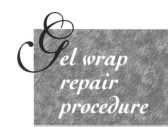

Gel wrap repair procedure

The gel wrap procedure combines the use of both of the systems. Supplies include fiberglass system, and a one-layer gel system plus the usual service supplies. If you use a multilayer system, ask the manufacturer which gel layer to use.

1. Cleanse the nail plate.

2. Glue the break closed. This is important. Shape the nail, as desired.

3. Remove the oils from the nail plate, then apply a base layer of the fiberglass resin.

4. Place a fiberglass strip horizontally into the resin and allow the strip to become completely saturated. Spray or brush on the activator. (Some technicians do not activate here, believing the fibers will disappear more.)

5. Apply a thin second layer of resin, apply the activator, then buff it a bit.

6. Apply a thin layer of gel as an overlay right over the resin/wrap and cure it as directed. The gel should be slightly beyond the wrap on the nail.

7. Apply a thin second layer and cure.

8. Finish the nail as the gel system suggests and proceed with the manicure.

Figure 3-7

Artistic designs can add a nice touch to special occasions.

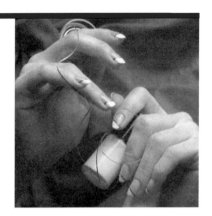

areas that are waxed that have this step. The waxing will perform the prep.) Clients love the convenience, and the soothing hydration performed immediately after the waxing during the manicure makes the pre-manicure timing perfect.

Some states permit this service to be performed by manicurists on the hands and feet, others are adding it as time passes. After all, it is within the licensing area of the manicurists. What a great service for a client who is annoyed by this condition!

Spa professionals and their employers must know the state regulations and perfect the skills for performing waxing services before adding these services to the nail spa menu. In most states, however, this service can only be performed by an esthetician or cosmetologist and the skills are only offered to the students in these specialty areas.

The addition of this allowance and the requirement that it be taught in the nail schools is a trend, but is controversial within our industry; those already licensed to perform this service are fighting it all the way to the licensing board and, many times, in the discussions before the legislatures.

Several reasons exist for the resistance to the addition of the skill to our service allowances, and most are legitimate concerns, as follow:

1. Waxing is not a technique taught to manicurists in schools. Those who are not trained will join those who are trained in offering the services. Important sanitation and damage precautions must be followed when performing this procedure.

2. Many manicurists will expand their service offerings beyond their areas of licensure ("to the knee and to the elbows"), such as to the face, bikini, and other sensitive body care areas. These areas must be appropriately, carefully, *and differently* treated than the areas allowed in the license for spa manicurists. The cautions are more stringent and the possibility of permanent damage is higher.

3. Many waxing services require a private area for performance of the services, which many salons do not have.

4. Cosmetologists and estheticians wish to keep this highly productive service to themselves.

The states, however, have some very good reasons for expanding this service into the license area of the manicurist, as follows:

1. The nail license needs more options for the menus of nail salons and departments to make them more profitable.

2. The nail client who is already sitting at the table likes the convenience of having her arms waxed or those few pesky hairs on her hands removed, right then, instead of having to move to another professional.

- Drop-ins and sample treatments—We are familiar with hot mitt treatments, paraffin dip treatments, and reflexology massage when they are done as "quickies." When these services are offered as samples, the prices for the regular services in which they are routinely included should always be mentioned, as well as their benefits, how long the service takes, and a suggestion for making an appointment,

Quickie and added-value services are limited only by the imagination of the spa manicurists. Wise spa professionals and menu designers think about what can be done in 15 minutes for waiting clients. Then they use these services to entice new clients to the nail spa from other areas of the salon. They provide great introductory opportunities or add dollars to the bottom line of the spa professionals and the nail spa!

This list is by no means all inclusive. The services and treatments should fit all the needs of the particular clientele of the salon, and the professionals will recommend them to meet those needs. They should be attractively described on the menu of services.

The old traditional menu of five items (new nails, fills, repairs, and basic and hot oil manicures) are gone for salons that want to build their clientele and add to the financial success of the nail professional and the nail spa. New and interesting products are being developed for expanding our services. As more products are formulated and available for nail spas, spa manicurists will develop wider capabilities for treatments and manicures, even though their licensing may not change, and menus will get larger and more interesting to our clients.

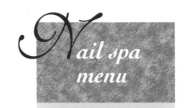

Nail spa menu

A balanced menu for a nail spa will have short and long services, medium-to-high cost services, and manicures, treatments, and enhancements. Its contents will be restricted only by the knowledge and imagination of the professionals.

Enhancements—Yes or No?

A controversy surfacing in the spa industry is whether or not acrylic enhancements should be a service offered in a spa. Those on the 'nah' side believe the odors caused by acrylic monomers are 'not spa,' while those on the 'yeh' side are adamant that these clients must be serviced in the spa or they will be lost to another business that will offer the service. Both sides of the controversy have a legitimate basis for their concerns and decisions. However, offensive odors *do not* have a place in spa concept salons. No matter how accustomed we are to them and feel they 'smell like money,' they must be dealt with in nail spas or they will adversely affect business. Spa clients *are* offended by these odors. After all, they pay more to come to a nail spa that *does not* offend them, either through odors or any other aspect of their service. However, I also feel that they can be dealt with efficiently to allow those clients to be serviced in the salon.

One of the problems in dealing with this issue begins with the spa designers. This can be a logistical and design nightmare unless the *primary* spa designer is informed of the problem *before he puts pen to paper*. Sad to say, however, many salon and spa designers are poorly informed and do not seem to understand the congruence of ventilation control and spa concept service. Even sadder, I have yet to see a nail spa that is large and beautiful—and designed by some guru salon designer who had no clue about spa concept—that has dealt with this problem perfectly. It seems always to be a problem! Spa clients with natural nails are seated right next to a client who is having acrylics applied, and more times than not will be offended.

No one has come up with a perfect solution for this problem, though there are adequate ones. Some decisions might be:

- *Absolutely perfect ventilation*—This nail spa will spend a ton of money on their ventilation to control the odors from acrylics. If the system works, no odors are discernable when a client walks in. The problem arises because the fumes that cause acrylic and other odors may not be well controlled between the tables in the nail spa, even though they are controlled well overall. A robed and relaxing client with natural nails who is annoyed with acrylic odors will at times be seated at the table right next to a client getting an acrylic application or fill. The fumes will greatly diminish the effects of spa concept service the client is experiencing. Her annoyance may be verbalized on her client survey, or even worse, she may discuss it with her best friend, who will discuss it with another friend, who…. The space between tables in the nail spa design is important in this situation. Local ventilation control can aid an overall ventilation system in improving the control of the fumes and odors.

- *Separate room* — Some spa concept salons have two areas for nail services — one where acrylics are done with a highly controlled ventilation and one where they are not. Never are clients with natural nails serviced in an area where acrylic odors are present in a salon that has made this decision and investment. (Fig. 3–8)

- *Gels and wrap focus* — Many nail spas have chosen to focus on gels and brush-activated wraps to alleviate the acrylic monomer odors completely. They may offer acrylics in a highly controlled area for clients who request them, but if a client comes in for new enhancements, gels or wraps are suggested, not powder and liquid acrylics. Other salons just go to gels and wraps, totally; no acrylics are applied at all. When a client with powder and liquid applications calls, she is told this and is offered the service they have chosen to focus on, but no monomer acrylics are offered.

- *Nonodor acrylics* — Some nail spas have gone to non-odor powder and liquid acrylics as a method of dealing with the acrylic odor situation. However, these products require a totally different acrylic application technique than traditional

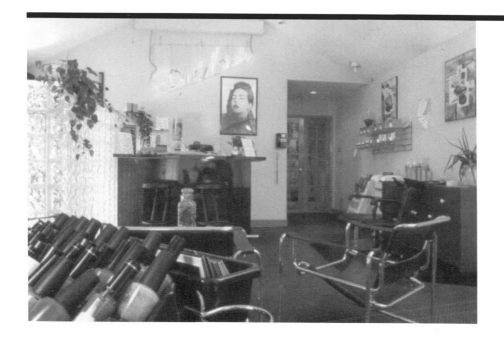

Figure 3-8

Separate rooms are set aside for clients applying acrylic nails.

acrylics and require new thinking on the part of the spa professionals to make them work. When this is accomplished, with training and practice, these products can be effective and the clients can be pleased with their results. When the salon does not bother to do this, their use can be a disaster.

- *Natural nails, only*—Some day spas do only natural nails in their nail spa. Their decision usually reflects a philosophy, and they will usually offer only skin care and body care— no hair services or acrylics are offered on their menu. (They are 'unnatural.') This is a 'niche' decision. The owners have decided that the cost of losing those clients will be bypassed by attracting their niche clients.

Whatever the decision for a nail spa concerning the offering of powder and liquid acrylics, it is a costly one. If the nail spa opts to offer powder and liquid acrylics, they are also opting for an expensive ventilation system, if it is to be effective at all, and some clients will still complain. If separate rooms are the decision, costly design and logistical problems will surface, although the cost will be much less if they are dealt with during the salon design stage rather than later. If only gels and wraps are done, a 'no service' cost is there—those clients will go elsewhere. If no acrylics are done, including gels and wraps those clients will go elsewhere, also.

This aspect of menu and salon design is a serious one for an owner. The wise owner investigates the situation, makes the decision, and makes the relevant design changes.

CHARGING APPROPRIATE FEES FOR MANICURES

The pricing schedule for individual services is important to the profit of the salon. Technicians and salons tend to charge low prices for manicures because of past poor service results; perhaps they subconsciously feel their manicures are not worth as much as other services, so they charge accordingly. The object is to *make the manicures "worth something" to the client*, and then, to *charge appropriately*. With this philosophy, manicures will be capable of producing a good financial return for the salon and professional. A client will only pay for a service that produces results she can appreciate as worthwhile.

This level of worthiness and profitability can be attained by upgrading the services and subsequently raising prices. Fortunately, new products and training are available to enable us to do this. If a nail professional learns and integrates new skin care-based manicuring methods, her service prices can be raised. The addition of these new skills, new professional and home care products, and a new attitude can make manicures fun as well as profitable.

One may define manicure fees by comparing them to other services and the units of time they take within the salon. Compare the price of a basic salon service that is equal in time to the basic manicure service; the price of the manicure should be the same as that basic service, assuming, of course, that the manicure is of appropriate quality. For instance, a salon may book out a half hour for a basic haircut, as it does for the salon's new basic manicure (not the old basic); the new basic manicure should have the same fee as the basic hair cut.

It may be difficult to raise prices in salons where the manicure has been low priced and producing poor results. In such circumstances, a compromise to circumvent this vision by the client might be made; the present water-based manicure service can be called an express manicure with the price retained, whereas the *new* basic manicure can be a new, more cost-equivalent price, meaning equivalent to the corresponding basic service in the hair department. The benefits of the new basic will be explained to each client during a sample appointment, and she will see the benefits for the upgrade on her own hands and nails. More on implementation is discussed in Chapter 15.

Treatment manicures should be scheduled for more time, and thus, cost more. To figure the charges for these more complex services, the following five points should be considered:

1. *The time that will be taken in the appointment book.* Most salons define a 'unit' of time as 15 minutes, probably because that has always been the way appointment books have been designed. If a service takes half an hour, that service is two units. The basic manicure needing a half hour will be priced as two units. The amount the salon charges for each unit will cover the overhead and the expected profit for the salon.

   Let's assume $20 as the price this salon expects for a half hour service, an easy figure to deal with and a common cost for a basic manicure in an upscale salon or nail spa. The hydrating manicure in this particular salon takes 15 minutes longer than the basic one so is half again longer than the basic. One half of the fee for the basic is $10. For that reason, the cost of the hydrating manicure should be, theoretically, $30.

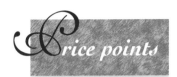

Price points

The viewpoints of the purchaser on those price points must be considered in choosing a charge for a service.

2. *The expertise required*. A manicure that requires extended training and expertise should cost more than the manicure equivalent in time. An example would be the exfoliating manicure that requires special training and discernment. If a basic manicure costs $20, an AHA exfoliating manicure of one hour should be $42 to $45, whereas an AHA exfoliating treatment may be $25 and one half hour. (See Chapter 5 for the difference between the two services.)

3. *Special or expensive products*. Few manicures require high cost and abundant products, but this is a consideration for some. A manicure that would fit into this category would be the exfoliation manicure because AHA systems are expensive.

Cost accounting a service can be complicated and time consuming because one spa professional will use more or less product than the next and take more or less time. For that reason, overall use can be a good decision tool. During the practice times, ask several testing spa professionals to mark their own bottle. They are the only one to use that bottle. They are also to keep track of the number of clients they do with that product. At the end of each bottle, the number is recorded and the figures used in an *approximation* of the costs.

Another method is to record the amount of a product used professionally over time (bottles), such as a year, and divide by the number of clients served. This method is probably reasonably accurate.

Using these methods, the overall cost of a product per service can be determined or at least a closer estimate can be made rather than guessing.

4. *Price points*. In our world, we see $29 as being a great deal lower than $30. It is not, at the worth of the dollar these days, but clients *see* it as being a lot lower than it really is in a dollar-to-dollar mental comparison. Conversely, some consumers may see a $31 charge more favorable than the $30 charge. (The $0 has much more negative effect on these clients than the $1 or $2.) The same effect is seen by us as consumers on the $35 price point versus the $34 and $36, though the viewpoint is not as definitive. For that reason, many salons will never price something on the $0 or the $5. For instance, that $20 upscale manicure is probably going to be $19 or $21, not $20, and the $30 manicure is probably $29 or $31.

5. *Prices based on the competition.* Many salons and day spas believe that they must base prices on their competitors'; their bottom line suffers from their lack of investigation and implementation. This method is not necessary if the salon's expertise, sanitation practices, customer service, and reputation deserve more. A spa concept salon with knowledgeable and fully trained spa professionals who use and recommend high-quality products *can* charge more than their neighboring salons. The clients will sell their services for them and their bottom line will show the results of their upgrade to spa. Conversely, a nail spa cannot price itself completely out of the market in which it participates. The wise owner will choose a balance of all these considerations.

MATHEMATICS OF MANICURES

Can manicures be profitable for you? Many enhancement technicians feel they cannot afford to do manicures, perhaps because they continue to do the old basic and hot oil manicures at the old fees. An adequate monetary return for every service is essential to provide sufficient motivation for our efforts. Is it possible that doing manicures can be as profitable as enhancements and, therefore, as attractive to manicurists?

Let's do some simple business math using the national average prices for manicures and fills to answer our question. For a sample comparison, assume you are an experienced technician who routinely does a fill in 45 minutes and a basic manicure in 30 minutes, and the fees being charged are the average fees for the old basic in the salons across the country. (The new basic may or may not be a higher price; spa manicures will deserve higher fees.)

For comparison, we must fit both services, completed, into an identical block of appointment time. In this example, both services fit, completed, into one and one half hours; three manicures can be done in the same time as two fills. Using the national average of charges (Nailpro Gold Book, 1998), $15 will be charged for a basic half hour manicure, and $20 for a 2-week fill; this technician can do three manicures ($45 plus) or two fills ($40). Any added treatments or services with the manicure produces additional income although many take little or no additional time. For example, sloughing is an extra $5 to $7, and takes no additional time using spa techniques. In contrast, fills using traditional methods have little opportunity for add-on services that fit into the allotted time to bring in 'plus' income. The numbers tell us that this technician can certainly afford to do manicures, if they are spa techniques and if she is willing to learn the necessary skills.

To determine a spa's possibilities, apply this income analysis method to the manicures and fills. If the fills are 60 minutes and the most basic manicures are 30 minutes, both services will fit completed into 1 hour as one fill and two manicures. Using the national average in pricing, the salon basic would produce $30 plus add-ons and skin care retail; the fill would produce $20, plus occasional retail.

Sample Using National Average Fees for Manicures and Fills

	Time	Completed Time	Fees	Total
Basic Manicures = $15	30 min	1-1/2 hrs	$15 x 3	$45
Fills = $20	45 min	1-1/2 hrs	$20 x 2	$40
Basic Manicures	30 min	1 hr	$15 x 2	$30
Fills	60 min	1 hr	$20 x 1	$20

All skill times and prices can be arranged for 'fit' and the salon prices plugged in. A 1-hour, 15-minute fill and one half hour manicure technician means she will have to use five hours of appointments for both to 'fit' for the calculations. Four fills will fit into 5 hours while ten manicures will also fit. Plug in the amounts and check the results.

Plugging in the Fees

	Time	Completed Time	Fees	Total
Basic Manicure	_____	_____	_____	_____
Fills	_____	_____	_____	_____

This analysis method is for comparative purposes only; it does not mean a technician has to perform 10 manicures to make it work. It is only a method for determining whether the skill is worth adding to the menu as a client service. The results can be enlightening, especially if the manicures are of high quality and the prices reflect this. If they aren't, shouldn't some changes be made?

Thirty Minutes for a Basic Manicure

A 'new basic' manicure can be designed to take only a half hour for the following reasons:

1. One half hour is sufficient for a new basic manicure. It is a basic manicure with massage only to the hand and no add-on treatments. A client who needs more time should be appointed for a treatment manicure that will more readily meet her needs.

   If she is a new client with troublesome cuticles, she should be told that 'Your first appointment will get you started toward controlling your cuticles.' A treatment manicure is suggested for the next visit.

2. This is the 'base' manicure, not a treatment manicure. It is designed for healthy skin and nails.

3. If a technician takes more than a half hour on a basic manicure with no upgrades, she is dawdling or talking too much. She needs efficiency training.

My suggestion, however, may not fit the market or service philosophy of many nail spas. Alas, it may be against the very philosophy of spa concept for a particular nail spa. If so, the manicure designer must proceed according to what is best for its clients and niche. The nail spa professionals must design the times of manicures to meet the niche in which they choose to be.

ENHANCEMENT TECHNICIANS

If a technician prefers acrylics and cannot force herself to do manicures, she should not rush to close this book. First, she can consider offering the skin treatments to enhancement clients. Just because the clients are getting enhancements instead of manicures does not mean that they do not need (and want) the skin care treatments. Actually, a client who cares enough about the appearance of her nails to purchase and nurture enhancements will also want her skin to look soft and beautiful. She will probably need skin care treatments and they can incorporated into:

1. The acrylic service

2. An acrylic manicure, as discussed

3. A separately appointed treatment-only service

When adding a skin care service to clients' appointments, their skin needs are being met. The professional can learn how to do the servic-

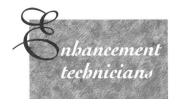

Enhancement technicians

Laura Massie, spa manicurist and nail technician, The Nail Spa at Golden Shears, Runnymede, NJ

I started doing nails 11 years ago, doing mostly acrylics and an occasional traditional "soak" manicure. Although I love doing nail enhancements, it can get pretty monotonous after awhile. I was getting burned out doing the same thing over and over. Then, we were introduced to the Spa Manicure.

"Spa Manicure" has brought variety to our nail business. It's a challenge because its something new, and because the clients are responding in such a positive way. Before they mostly ignored the skin care of the hands and arms, but now can't wait to book their next appointment. They not only want beautiful nails, but beautiful skin on their hands and arms, and the feeling of relaxation they enjoy during the experience.

These feelings of satisfaction have generated excitement for me, the client, and the entire nail salon. No more burn out for me!

The best part about Spa Manicure is that it does not only apply to the natural nail client, it is also for the nail enhancement client. I can't begin to tell you how much fun I'm having doing all the new spa manicures and treatments and anticipating the next one. Last week was the most fun work week ever in my 11-year nail career, and next week may be even better!

es, tell her about them, show her how well they work; the client loves the results! The salon incorporates the services into the service menu and appointment times, and the salon and professionals get a raise. Everyone's happy!

DOUBLE STATION TECHNIQUE

The professional who is booked with back-to-back appointments may see no way to add the spa concept to her schedule. In our industry, there *is* a glass ceiling that is at the limits of time and space the professional has available. What does she do? She adds a side nail table to her work area and her table becomes a double table set-up. Now she's on her way to a new level of income, with no more time in the salon, just more clients who are enjoying great spa treatments.

This new height in productivity can be done with double table technique. With a second table set to her right or left, this veteran can meet her client's needs while still allowing a relaxed atmosphere and service enjoyment for her clients. (See 'Double Station Technique' Fig. 3–9)

Double table technique is a system for working with two tables at the same station. It is fun for both the technician and the clients, and it is profitable. It is busy, but no more demanding or fatiguing than sitting at one table, if done properly. Actually, it can remove some of the stresses, such as running late, when one table does not allow the flexibility to overcome these problems.

The key to maintaining a pampering atmosphere and keeping the stress level down in double table technique is the professional's ability to maintain a client- care orientation. She must only change to a new client at the second table when the first client is in 'down time,' such as when she is scrubbing or in a treatment

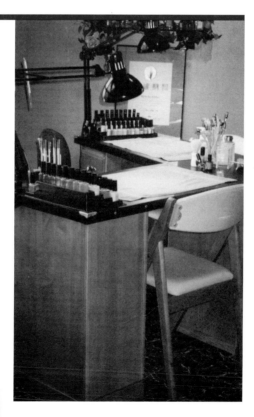

Figure 3-9

The Double Table technique allows for an enjoyable atmosphere for the clients and added income for the professional.

63

mode. (The professional moves, not the client.) It can be done, with a professional demeanor and client-care orientation. For instance, if an enhancement client is in for a treatment before her acrylic service, she is set up for the treatment while the professional's last client is washing and reappointing. Her treatment is started and she is relaxing in her treatment while the last client is being polished and released. After that client is released, the treatment client is ready to be prepped for her acrylic service. No time is wasted, and the client has had her wonderful and relaxing skin treatment. She's relaxed, and her skin looks wonderful right along with her nails when she leaves!

This technique is simple to do, but the professional must do it smoothly and in a pampering mode or it will fail, taking spa concept with it. It is ideal for the enhancement professional, however, who wishes to add spa treatments but has no added time to do so. If it is done properly, it is an option that can be wonderful for the client and profitable for the professional and the salon.

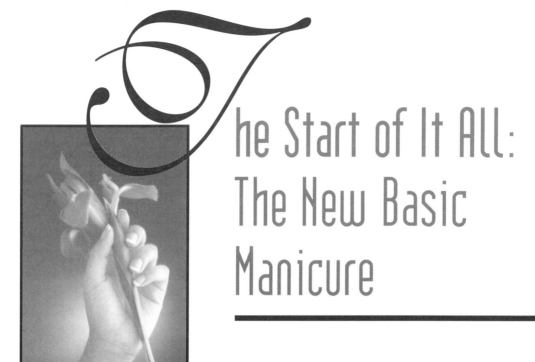

The Start of It All: The New Basic Manicure

4

OBJECTIVES

At the end of this chapter, you should be able to:

- State the differences between the traditional and new basic manicure.
- State the three reasons for removing water from the manicure.
- State the four advantages of the new basic manicure.
- State the three reasons for the new location for the massage in the manicure.
- Perform the new basic manicure.
- State the exceptions to the use of the water manicure and why.
- Tell your clients why you are doing a new type of manicure.

The spa manicuring technique begins with one pivotal manicure, a waterless, or oil technique manicure that becomes the basic manicure. The technique has always been available but we rarely used it; the water-soak manicure held the position of our basic manicure. However, this waterless manicure technique will soon exchange places with the traditional water/regular/basic manicure. It will become our new basic manicure while the water manicure will become the occasional manicure that we perform only under specific conditions.

Those few manicurists who have routinely used the waterless method for their basic manicure have chosen to do so for many (often not so good) reasons. Some use it simply because they do not have the time to prepare a water soak so they just skip this part of the manicure. They place oils or cuticle softeners on the clients' cuticles and start the routine from there. Others use the same procedure, but they do it because they do not like what water does to the nail plate. A few have completely reorganized the manicure procedure for the same reasons I have.

There are two important and obvious differences between the traditional basic and the new basic manicure. One is the removal of water as a part of the manicure routine (other than the client scrub at her entrance to the salon), and the second is the change in the order of the manicure to that similar to skin care: the massage is early in the manicure. The resulting evolution of the procedure takes manicuring far beyond that of the old basic. Because of these major differences, the only similarities between the new procedure and the prior water basic will be its placement on the salon menu as the basic manicure.

Several questions will be asked by the manicurist:

1. Why are we removing water from the regular manicure?

2. What is the advantage to this manicure?

3. Why is the massage at a different location in the service?

The explanations are revelations to us and change our way of viewing manicuring procedures.

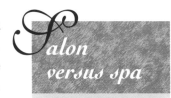

Salon versus spa

Suzie's Place
- Basic Manicure
- "Hot Oil" Manicure
- (Paraffin)

Suzie's Salon and Day Spa
- Basic Manicure
- Spa Manicure
- Basic Pedicure
- Spa Pedicure
- (Paraffin)

Elegance Nail Spa
- Spa Manicure
- Hydrating Manicure
- Aromatherapy
- Salt Glow Manicure
- Exfoliating Manicure
- Add-on Treatments
- Packages Available

WHY ARE WE REMOVING WATER FROM THE MANICURE?

We remove the water soak from the manicure, for several reasons. The first is the inherent design of our fingernail. A fingernail is constructed in overlapping layers, appearing similar to fiberboard. The layers

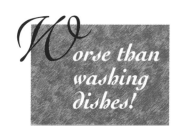

are held together by intercellular adhesive materials that make the nails into healthy and "hard" nails. When subjected to a soak, these oils and natural adhesives may be damaged or removed (at a minimum, a softening occurs), allowing the nails to be susceptible to damage and often causing a condition we usually refer to as *layering* or *peeling*.

How can a soak cause layering? Water is referred to by scientists/chemists and other experts as the universal solvent. Water will do the job when many other solvents will not. The situation is aggravated by the addition of some products to further soften the cuticles (detergent, in many situations). The natural adhesive in the nail plates is attacked by these solvents that can cause damage, which results in layering.

A second reason for not soaking in water, is the effects on the retention of polish. When a client's nails are soaked, the water is absorbed into the nail plate. In doing so, the nail changes shape; it relaxes, becoming more 'flattened' with less of a curve from side to side. This shape is retained for the most part, for the duration of the manicure, during which time polish is applied and dries.

Polish is a form of acrylic and hardens into the shape of the surface to which it has been applied, in this case the flatter nail plate. Later, the nail dries out and returns to its inherent shape, a curve from side to side, often damaging the retention of the polish. At best, there is a "pull" on the part of the polish in an attempt to return to its original shape, making it more susceptible to chipping and peeling. For this reason, those of us who prefer waterless manicures feel that polish lasts longer with the new no water method than when the nails are soaked.

THE ADVANTAGES OF THIS MANICURE

We would like our procedures to produce better results than our competition and differentiate us from them in a positive way. The new manicure system does just that for the following reasons:

- The entire hand will receive an intense softening treatment with this manicure. This is not true with the "fingertip soak" of the water manicure or with the lotion fingertip soak during the traditional hot oil procedure. The professional's focus is now expanded from just the nails to include the client's full hands.

- The skin care-based procedure produces *immediate* improvements in the skin because of the skin preparation for the treatments and the high quality of the products that meet the special needs of the client. This improvement will be easily noted by the client, and home care recommendations will maintain the service and continue to improve the skin and nails. The lotions are massaged in with a deep massage that will give a rosy, healthy look to the skin.

- The new basic defines a healthy, spa approach to a manicure. The water and hot oil manicures at other salons will seem a weak replacement to this manicure.

- This manicure is a different and more efficient routine than the basic one taught in beauty school. Once learned, this new procedure takes less time than the previous basic. When the manicurist becomes proficient with this manicure, she will do the procedure more rapidly than the regular water manicure in addition to providing the client with a more relaxing and therapeutic service.

Why Is the Manicure Procedure Different?

The manicurist has a different procedural order than the old water soak manicure. The noticeable change will the timing of the massage. The massage is *before* the cuticle treatment instead of after, and many of the treatments are *after* the massage rather than before. This procedure is similar to skin care services and is done for the same reasons.

First, the earlier massage stimulates the lower layers (dermis) of the skin to bring the natural moisturizers into the layers closer to the surface of the skin (epidermis) early in the treatment.

Second, the warmth of the massage opens the pores in the epidermis and increases the blood flow in the dermis. This allows a deeper penetration of the treatments, nutrients, and softeners, increases the provision of nutrients from the blood, and enhances the removal of toxins from the area.

The third advantage of the early massage is that it encourages the flow of blood to the fingertips and fingers. The nail matrix and cuticles are flooded with nutrients and moisture, which stimulates sluggish growth and moisturization, and cold fingertips feel warm, allowing the client to enjoy the warmth of her manicure.

The final advantage of the early massage is that it relaxes the client early in the service, allowing her a longer respite from her stressful world.

THE NEW BASIC MANICURE PROCEDURE

The client will be won over or lost during the first few minutes of the first appointment. Be professional, carry through the entrance routine, and welcome her with a smile. Most of the time, her first manicure will be the salon basic.

The new basic manicure is the skin care-based replacement for the traditional water basic manicure. Without "toots and whistles," it is designed for the client who does not need or want them. Her cuticles are healthy and intact, her nails are healthy, and her skin is normal. Following is the procedure for the new basic manicure.

1. *Entrance and seating of the client according to the procedure set by the salon.* A new client will fill out the salon information form before being seated. The preservice hand scrub will then be taught for a new client, according to the salon's procedure; a repeat client will proceed to scrub prior to seating (see Chapter 13). (Fig. 4–1)

2. *Client analysis.* Manicure and treatment recommendations are made during this step, and client choices are made. Home care and reappointment recommendations are discussed. (Fig. 4–2)

3. *Remove the polish and shorten/shape the nails.* This step is often integrated into the analysis step. Any large, loose, and obvious cuticle will be removed at this time to allow more efficient softening of the other cuticles; *no live tissue is removed.*

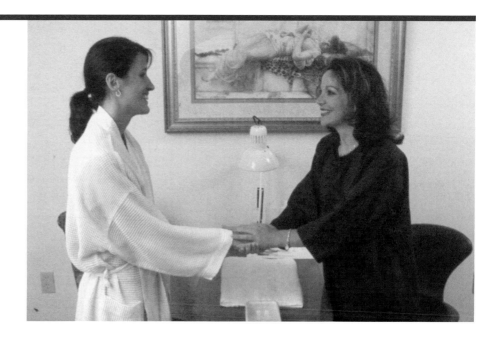

Figure 4-1

The first step is greeting the client.

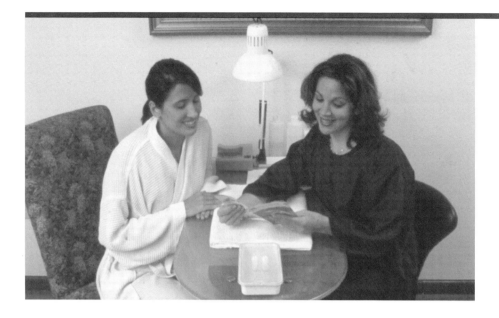

Figure 4-2

Client analysis enables the recommendation of services, home care, and future re-appointments.

4. *Hand massage*. The proper lotion is applied in a deep massage technique. The writing hand is massaged first, a cuticle treatment is applied, and then the hand is wrapped neatly in a towel (a dry, warmed one, if possible) and laid aside to allow the lotions to work. The procedure is completed on the second hand (see Chapter 6). (Fig. 4–3)

5. *Cuticle treatment*. After massaging and wrapping the second hand, the covering on the first hand is opened leaving the arm wrapped. Any remaining lotion and cuticle treatment are massaged in and a cuticle procedure is done. As the procedure is completed, a cuticle treatment is reapplied and the hand is laid aside to allow the treatment to work again.

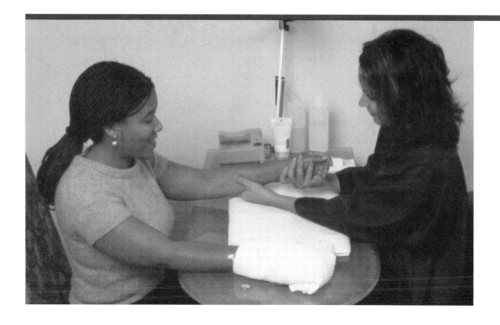

Figure 4-3

A cuticle treatment is applied and the hands are wrapped in towels.

(The hand is not wrapped.) The procedure is repeated on the second hand and it is laid aside. The first hand is now ready for "recheck" of the cuticle step (any wayward cuticles will have become apparent for removal) after which the second hand is rechecked for errant cuticles. An emollient cuticle oil is then massaged into the cuticles of both hands (avoid the nails).

6. *Nail bed cleansing/polish prep.* This step keeps polish on longer. First, use cosmetic-grade acetone to remove any debris and oils from the nail bed, carefully, keep it away from the skin and cuticles. Next, apply nail plate dehydrator, the one used to dehydrate and sanitize the nail plate before applying enhancements. This removes the oil from the outer surface, allowing the polish to adhere. (Using the new one-step nail plate cleansers/dehydrators eliminates one step.) (Fig. 4–4)

7. *Appointment "close" procedures.* These procedures, such as money, keys, appointments, and so on should be pleasant and routine. The table is cleared and cleaned in preparation for the polish step. Her keys are laid out and her money paid so that her polish will not be damaged. Her jewelry is replaced. Her coat is put on. Her appointment is made and the card placed in her purse. Her retail products are placed in a bag at her side. She is seated and made comfortable again. *Now* you can polish. (In large salons and spas, reappointments and service payment are as the client leaves, after the polish is dry.) (Fig. 4–5)

Figure 4-4

Applying a nail plate dehydrator removes oil from the surface, allowing polish to adhere longer.

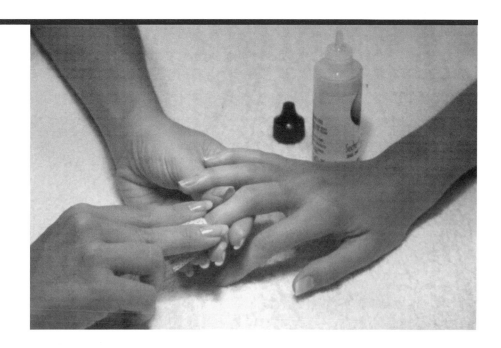

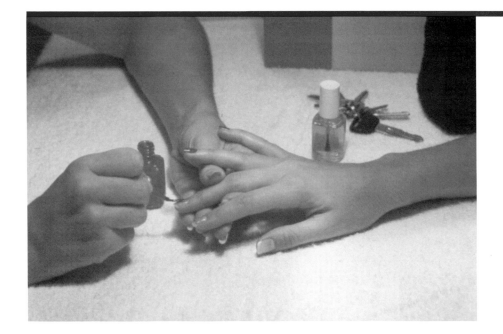

Figure 4-5

The polish application is the last step that takes place.

8. *Polish.* While you polish, all home treatments that have been suggested and sold must be discussed again, even though you have gone over them during the manicure. Her program is discussed in terms of what you may do at her next appointment, her home care regimen, and the results she will see at meeting her goal. If she is not on a program, her needs are discussed as well as the necessity for her to return and why.

9. *A drying procedure is ALWAYS performed.* Clients hate to wait for their polish to dry. For that reason, a spa manicure always includes application of a good quick-dry top coat and the requirement that she wait at least 3 to 5 minutes (whatever the drying product requires).

There are three reasons to use a polish dryer, even if it is not needed for the final result of the drying product. First, the client will feel like she is doing "her job" in the procedure and second, she will (usually) sit with more patience because she thinks she must as a part of the dismissal routine. Third, she will be less likely to damage her polish if she is required to sit in one place with no movement. Seat her comfortably in a drying area, and say a fond goodbye, or escort her out according to nail spa procedures. (Fig. 4–6)

Many nail spas have a separate drying area or a separate table to accommodate the client during this procedure. (When they continue to sit at the manicurist's table, they are delaying the seating of a new client.) Whatever the nail

Figure 4-6

The client is less likely to damage her polish prior to leaving the salon if she uses a dryer.

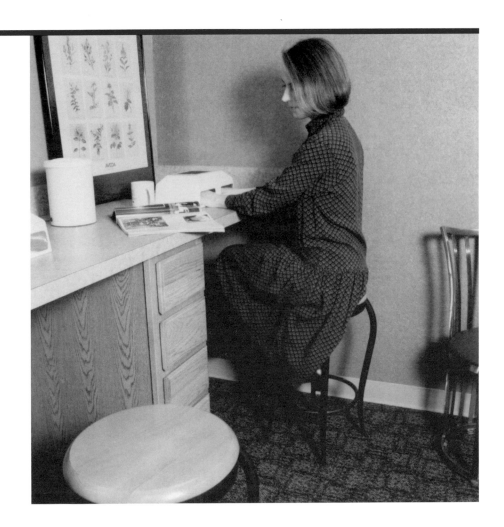

spa drying routine, the client should remain quiet for at least the amount of time the drying product recommends or she will require that dreaded, time-wasting polish repair.

10. *"Close."* Obvious sanitation procedures are performed in view of the client (see Chapter 13). Then, the table is made to appear as if no one has been there. Clients like to approach a station that is ready for *them*, not a station that is a visual reminder of its last occupant. Every nail spa should have an appointment closing routine that will accomplish this in less than 30 seconds. If a professional cannot do that at her station, she is working with too much clutter and needs to take a look at her lack of organization. Clutter does not support a spa atmosphere.

11. *Record keeping/computer work.* Most salon routines will require some type of record keeping after the client leaves. This is an important part of the service and should not be bypassed (see Chapter 12.)

Exceptions to the Rule

The nonsoak manicure is the basis for all the manicures in the spa manicuring system. The base philosophy of spa manicures and hand treatments is that nails are not soaked because of the potential harm it does to natural nails. There are four exceptions to that rule, however, though they are rare.

- *The client has nails so dirty or stained that the preservice scrub will not get them clean.* I doubt that many of these clients will be in a nail spa, but if they are, soak their fingertips in very warm water in a glass bowl, with an antimicrobial manicure lotion soap and a few drops of tea tree oil. Later, the soak bowl must be sanitized and the professional must be especially attentive to post-client asepsis practices. She must also take special care in her self-cleansing procedure after this client, scrubbing her hands and cuticles especially well with an antimicrobial hand cleanser. Her own health is an important consideration in this instance.

- *The client's cuticles are so sealed to the nail plate that soaking them is the only means that will encourage release for a manicure.* Usually this is a new client who has never had a manicure or at least not for an extended time, probably years. This client may be a chronic nail biter whose cuticles have become scar tissue.

  The client with overgrown and sealed cuticles can have beautiful cuticles with weekly manicures and dedicated home care. After this is accomplished, she too should be moved to waterless manicures.

- *The occasional client who wishes to have her nails soaked.* This client usually wants them soaked as they have always been, no matter the negatives to the water soak or the benefits to the skin care-based routine. Some clients are resistant to change and we must honor their request. When this happens, I suggest the professional soak the nails of one hand in a warm water and oil bath, *not a soap, shampoo, or detergent soak,* as she is massaging the other. If she can, keep the time to a minimum, then proceed with the service as usual. The service will be a little longer and the nails will be weaker, but the client is the boss, here.

- *The acrylic manicure requires a fingertip soak.* This is an acrylic brightening manicure and is discussed in Chapter 5. It should be done only on rare occasions because the brightener (Polident) will dry the client's skin.

Tell Them All about It

Most manicure clients have never experienced a manicure in which their fingers are not soaked. For that reason, the spa manicurist must explain to *every new client* why she is not soaking her nails. (Use the 'damaging to your nails' reason.) The explanation alleviates the chance of the uninformed client feeling she has been cheated, feeling that possibly the professional is shortcutting, or that she is doing the manicure improperly. Trust me…this is important. When I first switched to the waterless manicures, I did not explain what I was doing. One day, a client said to me, "My other manicurist always soaked my nails. Wasn't that better?" She had been having manicures weekly for years by another manicurist and was strong enough to come right out and ask me for the reason I was doing things differently. I explained my method to her and she was my client until I moved from that city.

That client's important question as was an awakener for me. I thought, 'What about all those other clients who hadn't asked?' From that day on I incorporated an explanation of why I would not be soaking her nails into my analysis of all new clients. It became a marketing tool to show the new clients how much better my manicure was going to be than others they had. I was careful, however, not to suggest that their other manicurist was wrong, merely to explain why this procedure was the one I did.

It is equally important that a spa professional provide a detailed explanation to her regular clients when she changes to this routine because they may see the new procedure as a "short cut." Most will come right out and ask, after we've held their hands for many appointments, they feel they can ask us anything. However, some will not ask and may go elsewhere to get the soak routine. For the transition of current clients, the "I-just-read-this-great-industry-book-that's-changing-my-way-of-doing-things" reason works well. Clients love hearing that their manicurist is striving to improve her techniques, especially those she uses on them!

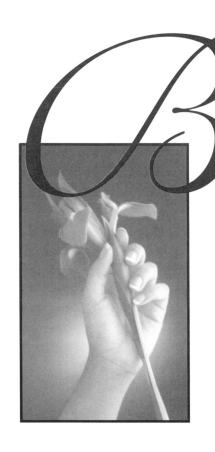

Beyond the Basics

5

OBJECTIVES

At the end of this chapter, you should be able to:

- Perform the spa manicure.
- Perform the hydrating manicure, hand facial, and paraffin treatment.
- Perform a sloughing treatment, exfoliating treatment and age-defying program.
- State the cautions for chemical exfoliation.
- Perform the nail growth program, matrix massage, and the grow off program.
- Conduct a nail biter program.

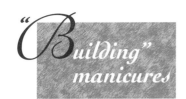

"Building" manicures

Spa manicures must always show their worth to the client in their results and pampering while allowing the spa to be compensated for the additional work and products being used. The manicures "build" on each other, allowing steps up in results and pampering while not making leaps past compensating the spa and professional for the work being done. The prices also build on the previous skilled manicures. Prices are determined by the costs, and the nail spa's niche.

Another basic advantage to designing manicures in a building sequence is that they are more easily defined by the learning manicurist. Examples are:

Basic—Traditional manicure in skin care order. It is the mini in a nail spa and the least expensive.

Spa Manicure—Basic manicure but has added the therapy and pampering needed for spa concept. In many nail spas, this manicure is the basic one. The price is higher than in the non-spa basic though it takes the same time as the above basic.

Hydrating Manicure—Spa manicure with skin preparation, heat mitts, possibly paraffin, or both, and a "sit" time. The time is at least 15 minutes more than the spa manicure, and the price is more. Treatment manicures start here in the building of manicures.

Aromatherapy Manicure—This is the hydrating manicure, with aromatherapy oils added in a synergy,

continued

Spa manicurists are state-of-the-art in skills, and the products they use in meeting the needs of their clients are the highest quality. They practice "prescriptive manicuring." They recommend treatments, manicures, and home care according to the conditions of the clients' skin and nails noted during the analysis. Their goal is to aid their clients toward improving their appearances and to pamper them in the process.

Successful spa manicurists always go beyond the basics in their client's care. Special services enhance their service menu, and they use the spa techniques chosen by their nail spa.

The new basic manicure is just what it indicates: a basic manicure for healthy and normal skin and nails. However, it is not "spa." *It will not improve the condition of the nails or skin.* For that reason, it must be upgraded in some manner to show some kind of improvement of the appearance of the skin and nails, even though they may be healthy and normal.

THE SPA MANICURE

Most nail spa clients will want more than the basics in their nail spa services. That is why they chose to go to a nail spa. For this reason, a spa manicure, a step up from the basic, is offered and the mention of it in the salon information indicates that it is "more than a basic" manicure. For instance, the spa manicure may be described in the menu as follows: *"Enhance the beauty of your hands and arms with our luxurious and relaxing spa manicure. Your hands and arms are treated and massaged with essential oil lotions that awaken the beauty of your skin. Your nails and cuticles are manicured and polished with the color of your choice."*

In the description of the basic manicure, the massage is described as being on the *hands only.* Essential oils or other upscale products and treatments are not mentioned. However, in the spa manicure, the treatments are described in pampering terms and include the arms—in some salons they specifically mention the elbows, also—bringing it beyond the basic category of service. An obvious differentiation must be seen in the descriptions to justify the upgrade in price from the basic manicure that clients will understand when reading the information.

Client Analysis

This client will want the extra pampering of the arm massage and the hydration of the spa of this manicure. She will have good skin, though it may be a little dry. Her nails can be normal or need treatment, as defined in the nail section of the analysis. The products used in this manicure will produce enhanced results because of the use of the skin products, the plastic encasement and possibly warmed towels.

Spa Manicure Procedure

This service is the new basic manicure with some added spa effects. First, the massage is performed on the forearm as well as the hand. Second, the hand and arm are placed in plastic wrap or thin baggies after the initial massage and placed in a towel or terry mitt. Last, towels are used as heat enhancers to produce enhanced penetration. (Fig. 5–1)

The "spa effect" of the plastic bag encourages the natural moisturizers of the lower layers of the skin (dermis) to come into the closer surface layers of the skin (epidermis). Further, the nutrients of the lotion will be more accepted into the warmed, open pores of the skin. The plastic wrap or baggies and towel are important to the spa effect. Following is a description of the spa manicure procedure, assuming that the manicurist understands the nuances of the steps that were described in the procedure for the new basic manicure. Only the differences between the new basic and the spa manicure are detailed.

1. *Entrance, preservice hand cleansing and seating of the client — according to the policy of the salon*
2. *Client analysis*

continued

as chosen by the client. The time allowed is the same as the hydrating, but the price is more.

Salt-Glow Manicure—This is the spa manicure with a physical exfoliation added. The time is the same as the spa manicure, but the price is more.

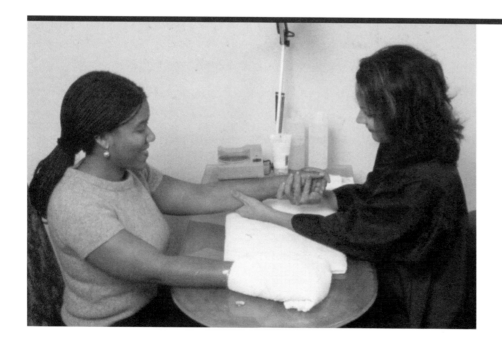

Figure 5-1

The new basic manicure utilizes some spa effects.

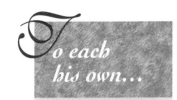

The manicures described in this chapter are not named with elaborate spa concept names because they may or probably should be in a nail spa's client information. Instead, they are named for their *function*, the basis for their inclusion on the menu in a nail spa. The appropriate name would be chosen by the menu designer, according to the salon ambiance, theme, and other criteria.

These manicures represent the basics of their function and design, (i.e., the hydrating manicure), and may be redesigned according to the product lines chosen and treatment criteria for the particular nail spas in which they will be used. These manicures merely scratch the surface of those that may be designed for the use of a good nail spa. They are, however, a great place to start!

3. *Remove the polish and shorten/shape the nails/remove obvious dry cuticle.*

4. *Hand and arm massage.* The spa manicure implements a spa effect after the massage of each hand and arm. (The new basic only massages the hands, then places them in a towel.) After the massage, additional moisturizer is applied to the hands and arms, essential oils are massaged into the nail plates to enhance "plasticization" of the surface of the nail, and cuticle lotion treatment is massaged into the cuticles to enhance the cuticle treatment. The hand and arm are placed in plastic wrap or a thin plastic bag, then wrapped in a towel and placed aside. To enhance the spa effect, a heated towel can be used, it desired. Each hand is left in the spa environment only while the next procedure is being performed on the other hand. No set time is implemented in this manicure.

5. *Cuticle treatment/ recheck*

6. *Nail bed cleansing/polish prep*

7. *Appointment close procedures*

8. *Polish applied*

9. *Drying procedures*

10. *Postprocedure sanitation activities*

Many upscale salons and nail spas use this manicure as their basic manicure, eliminating the non-spa basic manicure from their menu completely. They feel spa effect is important even in their very basic service and wish to set their lowest standard far above that of other salons.

Time Allowed

The appointment time for a spa manicure is an important decision for the menu designer. Following are some considerations:

Pricing

— A high ticket salon may charge enough for this manicure to be 45 minutes or more. If so, the massage can be lengthened.

— A moderate ticket salon must keep it at one half hour.

Treatment manicures

— The treatment manicures must be longer than this manicure.

The basic

— If this is the basic manicure of the salon, it should be moderate in time. If not, it can be longer.

Client perception

— The expectations of the clients should be considered, but not enough for the manicure to cease being profitable.

Profitability

— The time/price interaction should ensure that the spa and spa professionals can make money on the manicure.

Prepping the Skin for the Products

One of the main philosophies in skin care is that one prepares the skin for treatments. This preparation removes any barriers to the treatments from the surface of the skin to allow optimal acceptance of the products for doing its work. For instance, the surface oils, debris, and dead cells are removed before the application of a hydrating or exfoliating treatment. The treatment manicures and treatment procedures in spa manicuring incorporate this philosophy and usually begins in the first treatment manicure, the hydrating manicure, though some will begin at the spa manicure.

HYDRATING MANICURE

The spa manicure is the base service of this manicure. It is designed for alleviating dry skin through deep hydration of the skin and cuticles. This and other therapeutic manicures are especially beneficial for clients in a cold climate, though there are many other reasons for dry and dehydrated skin such as overexposure to the sun and other occupational and environmental factors.

Client Analysis

This client has dehydrated or dry skin and needs the extra moisturizing treatment of the hydrating manicure. Her nail treatment will be according to the spa manicurist's analysis.

Hydrating Manicure Procedure

This manicure is similar to the mitt manicure that is used in our industry at the present time, with these differences:

- The water soak is not used on the fingertips.
- The arm is included in the treatment.
- A skin preparation step is performed.
- The procedure is the new order.

Spa manicuring versus the "spa manicure"

Spa manicuring as a collective concept is a number of manicures that unite pampering, luxury, immediate results, rejuvenation, relaxation, and other aspects of being spa with analytical skills and knowledge that can enable a manicurist to meet each client's needs. A spa manicure, the basic manicure upgraded to spa, is a particular manicure that is performed within this concept. It is not usually a manicure that contains a mask.

The client sits for a time with both hands in the electric heat mitts with no additional service being performed by the spa professional. This should be a quiet time for relaxation and rejuvenation.

Stepping up to a skin care manicure procedure will enhance the effects of the treatment, and thus, its immediate and lasting effects for the client.

1. *Entrance, preservice client cleansing and seating of the client, according to the policy of the salon*

2. *Client analysis*

3. *Remove the polish and shorten/shape the nails/remove obvious dry cuticle*

4. *Skin preparation.* To enhance the absorption of the treatment ingredients, the skin must be prepared. First, remove the surface oils of both the hand and arm with a makeup remover and 4″ x 4″ squares that can be purchased where skin care products are sold, or with a physical exfoliating product (see Chapter 10). The skin prep is performed using dramatic effleurage movements that will draw the attention of the client to the procedure. (She needs to see it as a separate step from the massage).

5. *Deep hand and arm massage/set time.* The massage in a hydrating manicure is performed with a high-quality moisturizing lotion. After the hand and arm are massaged and placed in the plastic, the hand is placed in a thermal hand system (electric mitts) during the time the next hand is being treated; warm towels are a good choice for adding heat to the arms. The hands are left in the system 10 to 15 minutes, according to the wishes of the menu designer, which means there is a *set time* for the client during the manicure between the application of the lotions and the massage for the second hand and the end of the 10 to 15 minutes treatment time for

Figure 5-2

The client stays in the heat mitts for a designated time set by the salon.

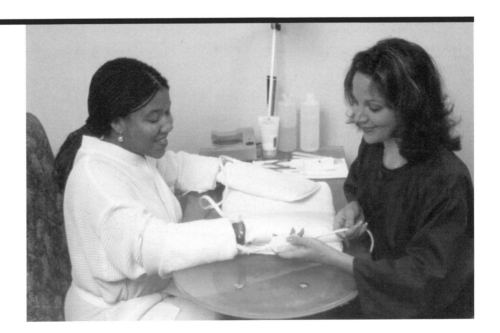

the first hand. (Fig. 5–2) The spa manicurist makes certain the client is comfortable for the few minutes she is sitting and leaves her to relax. The ambiance of the room should support this pampering time.

6. *Cuticle treatment/recheck.* At the end of the set time for the first hand, the hand is removed from the heat mitts and the plastic, and the cuticle treatment is performed. The cuticle treatment for the second hand is done after the first hand. (Usually the set time of the second hand is completed during the cuticle treatment of the first hand.) Leave the towels on the arms of the client during the cuticle treatment. (Many spas use long plastic bags to encase the hands and arms during the set time and will cut off the plastic bag at the wrist to enable the prolonged hydration of the arms during the cuticle treatment.) Recheck the cuticle after the treatments. An emollient cuticle oil is then massaged into the cuticles of both hands (avoid the nails).

7. *Nail bed cleansing/polish prep*

8. *Appointment close procedures*

9. *Polish applied*

10. *Drying procedures*

11. *Postprocedure sanitation activities*

- *Add-ons* — Paraffin can be added before the plastic bags and mitts.

- *Home care suggestions* — This client will need all the hydration she can get. Recommend a high-quality emollient hand lotion and an essential oil cuticle oil for generous use.

- *Future appointment recommendations* — Hydrating manicures with paraffin will be the manicures for a person with dry skin, plus hand facials and aromatherapy manicures. Exfoliating manicures will improve the texture of the skin and allow improved penetration of the emollient products.

Elbow Care

Many spa manicurists check the condition of the client's elbows during analysis because clients whose hands are excessively dry may also have very dry elbows. Many nail spas will include hydration of the elbows as a bonus service and do not charge extra unless a physical exfoliation is needed. Simple hydration is done by extending the application of the lotion onto the elbow during massage and extending the encasement of the plastic up past the elbow by using plastic wrap or the longer plastic bags (Fig. 5–3). (The prep step is extended to the elbow also.)

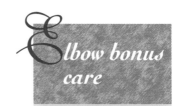

Elbow bonus care

Be certain the client knows this is a bonus service by mentioning it during the analysis, such as, "Oh dear, I need to do some extra hydration on your elbows, also. I'll do that before and after the hand and arm massage." Then do an elaborate (though short) application of a good hydrating lotion with the open palm of the hand— use of the fingers may affect the ulnar nerve, the "crazy bone," and cause the client discomfort.

Figure 5-3

Simple hydration can take place by extending the lotion past the elbow and following with plastic wrap.

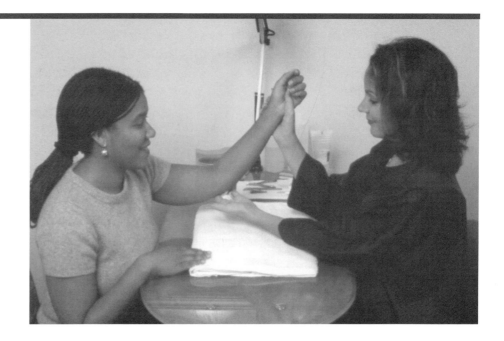

If exfoliation is needed, a separate physical exfoliation service before the hand and arm massage step should be performed and charged as an add-on, usually $3 to $7. No extra time is generally added to the service time for this add-on. Use an elaborate effleurage and a good exfoliating product that has a moisturizing lotion base. This product will have granules of some sort for performing the removal of the callused skin.

Removal of the exfoliating product should be simple and complete, allowing the massage lotion to be applied for hydration. The product can be removed with "exfoliating gloves," the scratchy nylon gloves sold for body care products, or by a towel.

Aroma-therapy manicure

The aromatherapy manicure is the signature manicure of "being spa!" It is relaxing, rejuvenating, and treating. For that reason, it is considered the "gift" manicure. When a person calls to purchase a gift, the receptionist suggests this manicure (and possibly the accompanying aromatherapy pedicure) as it is the one that is most relaxing for the one-time guest.

AROMATHERAPY MANICURE

This manicure is the hydrating manicure with the use of aromatherapy oils. It is designed to alleviate dry skin through deep hydration, but it is also considered highly pampering and rejuvenating due to the addition of the aromatic oils. It is a very popular gift manicure because it is very relaxing. Nail spas should suggest this to any person purchasing a gift due to its high "ahhhhhhh" production in the clients who have it.

Client Analysis

This manicure is for the person who needs the extra pampering and rejuvenation of the oils, although it is a highly moisturizing manicure for dry skin, also.

Aromatherapy Manicure Procedure

Because this manicure uses aromatherapy oils, during step 2 the client will choose her desired aroma from an offering of three. Two choices are not enough, and more than three are too many. Keep the decision simple. The theory of this choice is that the client's body will tell her which aroma she needs. However, do not make this a big deal by explaining the philosophy to her. Just wave the bottles for her to smell the aromas and ask. She does not want to make big decisions here. (Fig. 5–4). Then, the lotion, oils, and aromasols are chosen all with that same aroma—she is gently immersed in that enhancing aroma for her entire manicure (see Chapter 8).

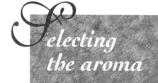

Selecting the aroma

When offering the oils for choosing, do not allow the client to see the names of the oils or she will choose them by name instead of by aroma. This can cancel their benefit. Suggest that she close her eyes, relax, and take a "cleansing breath" between choices.

1. *Entrance, preservice client cleansing and seating of the client, according to the policy of the salon.*
2. *Client analysis.* After the analysis, the client will be offered the three oils and she will choose the one she prefers. The lotion, oil, and aromasols will be retrieved for their use. Towels will be sprayed with the appropriate aromasols.
3. *Remove the polish and shorten/shape the nails/remove obvious dry cuticle.*
4. *Skin preparation.* To enhance the absorption of the treatment ingredients, the skin must be prepared. Either remove the natural oils with makeup remover or apply the chosen aroma oil to the skin, then perform the physical exfoliation with herbs or another product that can be used as an exfoliate with the oils. The skin prep is performed using dramatic effleurage movements that will draw the attention of the

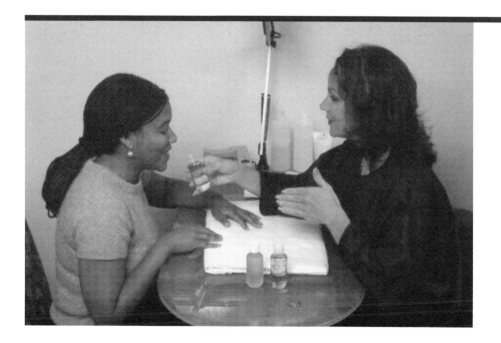

Figure 5-4

Gently wave the oil in front of the client so she is aware of the aroma.

client to the procedures. (She needs to see it as a separate step from the massage.)

5. *Hand and arm massage/set time.* Apply the chosen aroma lotion after the makeup remover or over exfoliating granules that will melt into the lotion. Perform a deep hand and arm massage, then place hands and arms in the plastic. The hand is placed in a thermal hand system (electric mitts) during the time the other hand is being treated. Warm towels that have been sprayed with the aromasol oils of the chosen aroma then heated are a good choice for adding heat to the arms, also, because of the aroma integration. This is the choice of the menu designer. The hands are left in the warming system 10 to 15 minutes, according to the wishes of the menu designer, which means there is a set time for the client during the manicure between the application of the lotions and the massage for the second hand and the end of the 10 to 15 minutes treatment time for the first hand. The spa manicurist makes certain the client is comfortable for the time she is sitting and leaves her to relax. The surroundings should be pleasant support this pampering time.

6. *Cuticle treatment/recheck.* At the end of the set time for the first hand, the hand is removed from the heat mitts and the plastic, then the cuticle treatment is performed with the aromatherapy oils. The cuticle treatment for the second hand is done after the first hand. Leave the aromatic towels on the arms of the client during the cuticle treatment. Recheck the cuticle after the treatments. The aromatherapy oil is then massaged into the cuticles of both hands (avoid the nails).

7. *Nail bed cleansing/polish prep*

8. *Appointment close procedures*

9. *Polish applied*

10. *Drying procedures*

11. *Postprocedure sanitation activities*

- *Add-ons* — Many nail spas will include paraffin in this manicure; it is applied just before the plastic bags.
- *Home care suggestions* — Many clients will purchase the aromatherapy lotion and oils for their home use. Suggest they use them generously for dry skin.
- *Future appointment recommendations* — Future appointments should be recommended according to the overall conditions of the client's skin and nails.

HYDRATING HAND FACIAL

This hyperhydrating skin and cuticle treatment can be done as a separate appointment to the manicure or as a manicure. It is a hydrating routine using products and the routine of a salon facial hydrating system, thus the name, or newly available products specifically packaged for a hand facial. The purpose is to deeply hydrate the skin. It is performed after as a alternate appointment to the sloughing manicure or the exfoliating manicure, or just as a treat to those who may be tired of the effects of the winter or sun on their skin.

This service takes time and adds up in price, even more so when it is a manicure. Most facial systems require cleansing, exfoliating, massage, a mask, and postmask hydrating. Systems specifically designed for hands, however, may be less complex.

The system designer should look at facial systems closely to see if they meet the needs of hands; the designer can choose one especially designed for hands or use individual products, such as those mentioned in the procedure below.

Client Analysis

This client has severely dry skin or just wants an intense pampering. This treatment can be especially effective for the client who has environmentally or occupationally dry skin and wants fast results. If there is chaffing, however, the prep step must be very gentle.

Hand Facial Procedure

If a facial or manicure facial system is chosen, the professionals will follow its treatment procedure. Following is a nonproduct line procedure.

1. *Entrance and seating of the client according to the policy of the salon*
2. *Client analysis*
3. *Remove the polish and shorten/shape the nails/remove obvious dry cuticle.*
4. *Skin preparation.* To enhance the absorption of the treatment ingredients, the skin must be prepared (the surface oils removed). The spa manicurist has several choices: cleansing with a facial quality cleanser that is included in a facial line, removing the surface barrier oils by use of a makeup remover or using a lotion physical exfoliator. The prep must be dramatic in the eyes of the client because this is an expensive treatment.

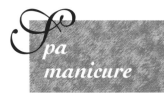

Spa manicure

The Hand facial is the procedure that many salons and spas offer as their "Spa Manicure," and mostly in the old order of procedure. In doing so, they are restricting the use of professional analysis by their manicurists, cancelling the other manicures from their menu, reducing therapeutic results and the income of the department. Most salons who do this have only two manicures, the basic and the spa manicure.

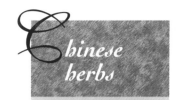

5. *Hand and arm massage.* The massage is performed with a moisturizing lotion. After the deep hand/arm massage, moisturizing lotion is reapplied to the arm and a treatment is applied to the cuticles. The hand and arm are placed in a plastic bag and a warm towel is wrapped around it. The second hand and arm are massaged and moisturized and placed in the bag and towels.

6. *Moisturizing mask.* After the massage of the second hand, the plastic bag is removed from the first hand and a moisturizing mask is applied according to the directions. The pre-mask encasement in the plastic enhances the treatment capabilities of the mask product by opening the pores. The hand is placed again into the baggie and set aside in warm towels. The same procedure is done to the second hand and arm.

   After the time indicated in the directions for the mask, the hand is removed from the plastic, and the mask is removed from the hand with warm, wet, aromatic towels. A moisturizing lotion and SPF 15 lotion is applied to the hands.

7. *Cuticle treatment/recheck*

8. *Nail bed cleansing/polish prep* (optional)

9. *Appointment close procedures*

10. *Polish applied* (optional)

11. *Drying procedures* (optional)

12. *Postprocedure sanitation activities*

- *Add-ons*—A mask for the arm can be offered as an upgrade for a client with dry skin in that area ($10-15). (Fig. 5–5) This increases the time and cost of the procedure, as well as the charges, and is a good service to those who need it. Always include the elbow in the masking of the arms; this client will need it.

- *Home care suggestions*—This client will especially need hydrating lotions and cuticle oils at home. A low AHA lotion is also good for her use. If she has no openings in her skin, a high AHA is important, applied once per day, plus an AHA cuticle treatment.

- *Future appointment recommendations*—Hydrating manicures will be wonderful for this client, with added paraffin in the mitts. Also, after any openings are healed, an AHA treatment series will improve her skin greatly.

Many nail spas will perform this as a treatment only, removing the nail plate services, to allow shortening the appointment time and to reduce the charge. This is a viable reduction because it is a concentrated treatment for the skin and cuticles that can be done separately from the nail

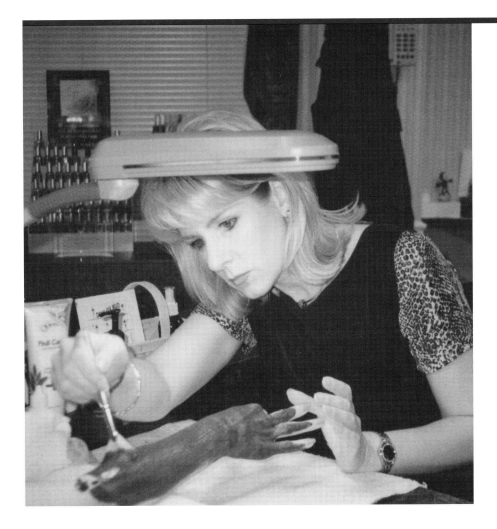

Figure 5-5

Upgrading can include
a mask for the arm.

plate treatments. This is the decision of the menu designer and management of the spa.

Many spas add paraffin to this treatment, applied immediately after the application of the mask, which increase the cost of the treatment, and, therefore, the fee the client is charged. The paraffin enhances the effects because of the heat and barrier qualities. This is a great treatment for the "winter blahs."

The time involved in this treatment is extensive, especially if paraffin is included, possibly 1 hour, most times more. The spa manicurists who perform this treatment must be well trained in efficiency of movement and time, and must stick tightly to the schedule. They must practice, practice, practice, and meticulous clock watching is the key. (The hair designers in the salon will need these treatments and are excellent practice clients.)

This is a high ticket treatment for the skin, but it shows great results. The charges will range from $35-$50, according to the time, the products used, and the niche of the nail spa.

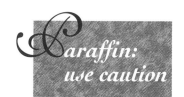

PARAFFIN TREATMENT

Paraffin has been used for years as a dip-and-heat mitt treatment. It feels wonderful and clients react well to it. The problem? It was a placator that only had minimal results. Although it feels great at the moment, the hands quickly return to their prior condition. For it to be a successful treatment, the skin must be prepped with a physical exfoliator before the treatment lotion is applied, then dipped in the paraffin and placed in heat mitts. It takes a few more minutes, but it is a much more effective treatment for dry skin.

Paraffin can be a separate treatment or part of another manicure, such as the new basic, spa, hydrating, hand facial, or aromatherapy manicures. Many spas will include paraffin in many of their manicures to ensure the results and to justify a higher price. This is the decision of the menu designer.

The treatment effects of paraffin are simple. The paraffin holds the treatment lotion to the surface of the skin, while the heat enables great penetration of it into the skin. The elastin and collagen fibers in the dermal layers of the skin are stimulated to regenerate by the heat and the product that is absorbed. The heat from the paraffin produces perspiration, which cannot escape the surface of the skin, so it is forced into the surrounding layers of the skin, plumping it up and providing hydration to the dehydrated cells.

Paraffin Procedure

Three options are available for location of application paraffin during a manicure. First, the application can be done after the massage. The lotion is reapplied, then the paraffin, to enhance its affects. Second, the paraffin can be applied after the cuticle treatment, just before the nail plate cleansing and polishing. Third, the paraffin can be applied after the polish has been applied and has dried for 3 to 5 minutes, but only if a very speedy quick-dry topcoat is used. The placement of the application is the decision of the spa manicurist.

After the paraffin application, the hand is placed in plastic, then into electric or terry mitts; a sitting time of at least 10 minutes is suggested. Then removal is accomplished by folding the paraffin and plastic bag toward the skin at the top of the applied paraffin. The "glove" is easily removed, bringing the paraffin with it. The remaining treatment lotion is massaged into the hands.

If the paraffin does not come off in a nice neat glove, it has not had enough lotion under it, has not had enough paraffin layers applied, or the thickness was uneven.

Sanitation Concerns

The traditional application of paraffin is dipping of the hands directly into the paraffin. However, some clients and spa manicurists have sanitation concerns about dipping their hands into a paraffin pot that has had repeated dips by prior clients. I will not discuss the validity or non-validity of this concern; I will suggest, however, that accurate or not, this client concern should be a consideration in choosing the procedure for the application of paraffin in a nail spa service.

One alternative application procedure that can be considered to accommodate this concern can be the application of the paraffin with cheesecloth or paper towels. The procedure is simple, though quite dramatic, which can be an advantage! Another advantage is that the paraffin does not feel as hot, as it does in a dip, although it is warm enough to feel wonderful. Also, the heat is retained longer with the cheesecloth or toweling. (Fig. 5–6)

The paraffin pot is brought to the client and placed next to her at the station. The lid is opened and laid, upside down, against the pot and leading toward the client. The lid catches any drips that might happen in the transfer of the cloth or toweling toward the client. (This lid will become a housekeeping issue because the drips left on it will be seen by clients.) Then, a pre-cut piece of cheesecloth that has been opened to its maximum size is dipped; the vertical dip is redone two to three times and the cloth allowed to drip for a few seconds. Next, the cheesecloth is transferred to the client and wrapped loosely, then pressed tightly to the client's hand. (Fig. 5–7)

Some spas use this method to add a paraffin treatment to the forearm and elbow, which are then encased in plastic wrap or a long plastic bag. If so, the spa professionals need to practice this several times or they will be very messy.

If paper toweling is used, use at least two sections of a very soft and highly absorbent toweling. Cheap paper towels will not absorb the paraffin nor are they crushable against the skin. Use the above-described method for application.

Another method for application is less dramatic. The plastic bag is crushed as we do with hosiery before putting a toe in it. The index finger and thumb of the professional's non-writing hand are placed together in an 'O,' then the bottom of the bag is pushed down into the O to become the basket that will hold the wax. (Fig. 5–8) One-third to one-half cup of paraffin is dipped out of the bath and into that little basket, the client's hand is pointed into the basket, and the plastic bag is pulled

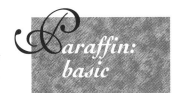

Paraffin: basic

Heather Sweat, from Just Imagine, Oak Ridge, Tennessee, had a difficult time upgrading her clients to paraffin from her basic manicure, so she added it into the new basic procedure as a part of the service. Also, it took too much time if it was added as an additional service, outside the manicure service. "I book every 45 minutes for acrylics, so my basic manicure has to be 30 minutes and be good enough to pull in enough to make it worth doing."

Her basic procedure is the new basic manicure with added paraffin, though she does let them sit a few minutes. "After my massage, I add cuticle remover, then dip the client's hands and let them sit 5 to 10 minutes—usually 5 is enough. Then I remove the paraffin and continue the manicure. The manicure takes 30 minutes and I charge more than the normal charge for a basic, because it has the paraffin treatment in it."

This upgrade to her basic has worked well for Sweat because no other salon around includes paraffin in the manicure. The clients love this basic manicure and are willing to pay the extra amount. Sweat loves it because she can easily get done in 30 minutes as the cuticles are well softened.

Figure 5-6

Alternatives to dipping into paraffin can be performed.

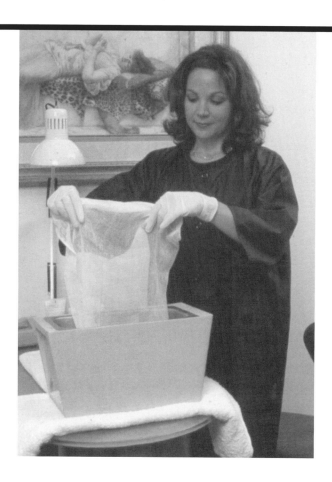

Figure 5-7

A piece of cheesecloth or paper towel can be used to apply the paraffin.

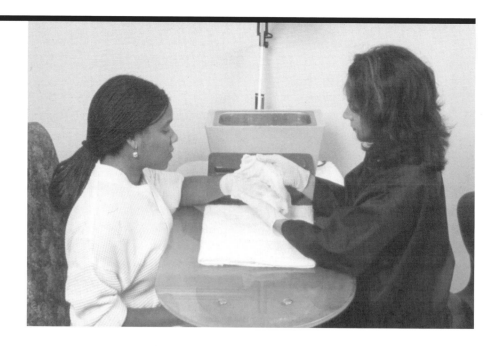

over the client's hand. (Fig. 5–9) (Do not try this with the large opening plastic bags from the hair department. I did and made a real mess.)

Next, the spa manicurist speedily manipulates the paraffin up around the client's hand and arm. The hand with the bag is placed in the mitts, and the client is encouraged to relax. This method is effective, though it depends on the thoroughness of the spa manicurist for coverage. It certainly is neater than the other methods, though it does take some practice. The wax is more difficult to pull off in a glove also due to the uneven coverage.

Estheticians often apply paraffin with a facial brush. The brush is dipped into the paraffin, then brushed onto the skin. It is slower and more tedious than the methods mentioned above, but is quite impressive.

SLOUGHING

Sloughing, or physical exfoliation, can be suggested as a separate treatment, a preservice treatment before another manicure, or a manicure service in itself, called a sloughing manicure. The manicure is a spa manicure with a sloughing treatment incorporated into the start of the massage. It treats the skin and cuticles of the client and is highly appreciated by those who need it. The product should contain gentle exfoliates, leaving smooth, moisturized skin after its removal. Many sloughers are available and include salt glow products, lotions with granule exfoliants, and herbs.

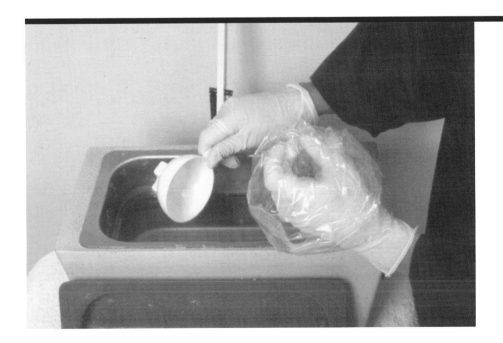

Figure 5-8

Paraffin is poured into a plastic bag held in a circle of thumb and finger.

Figure 5-9

The plastic bag is pulled
over the client's hand.

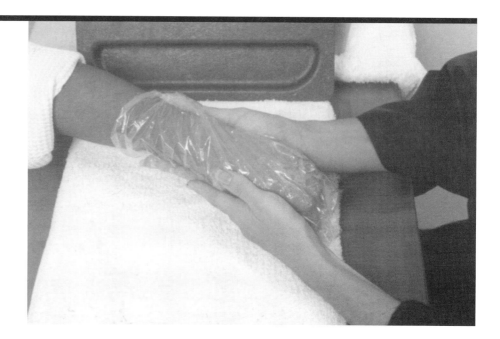

Salt glow is an exfoliating service that has become a sought-after treatment in the spa industry. Many spas have salt glow manicures, salt glow pedicures, and salt glow body treatments on their menus. The client's skin feels smooth and soft after a salt glow treatment, which incorporates wonderful hydrators in the service.

Client analysis

Sloughing is designed for the client who wants immediate relief from roughness on systemically, environmentally, or occupationally dry skin. She has dead cells on the surface and may have microscopic lesions or openings in her skin, so chemical exfoliation is not an option.

Sloughing Procedure—A Treatment

As a separate treatment, the sloughing product is gently massaged over clean skin until most of the lotion is absorbed, then the sloughing particles are removed with a cloth towel. (Salt glow works a little differently; read the directions for removal.) Usually, the treatment is carried up to and including the elbows. After the product is removed, the skin is additionally moisturized with the appropriate lotion; then the client is released.

Sloughing should not be the preparation treatment before chemical exfoliation because it might scrape the surface of the skin, producing minute scratches unless it is an extremely gentle physical exfoliator. The following chemical exfoliation can be uncomfortable and the mechanism for the workings of the chemical exfoliants interrupted. It is best to stick to the pretreatment preps that are recommended by the product line being used.

Sloughing Manicure Procedure

The usual base manicure is the spa manicure. The intensity of the dryness, possibly accompanied by chaffing on some clients, will be the basis of the decision. A lotion-based slougher is best over severely chaffed skin because salt glow may be uncomfortable. The following procedure is sloughing within the spa manicure.

1. *Entrance and seating of the client according to the policy of the salon*
2. *Client analysis*
3. *Remove the polish and shorten/shape the nails/remove obvious dry cuticle*
4. *Sloughing/deep hand and arm massage.* Physical exfoliation should be performed before the deep hand and arm massage with gentle effleurage movements. It there is a residue, remove it with warm towels or a sloughing glove, the prickly nylon gloves sold in body care shops. After the sloughing and massage are performed, the hand and arm are placed in plastic wrap or a thin, plastic bag and placed in mitts. Each hand is left in the spa environment only while the other hand is being worked on in the last or next step; usually 5 to 10 minutes.
5. *Cuticle treatment/recheck*
6. *Nail bed cleansing/polish prep*
7. *Appointment close procedures*
8. *Polish applied*
9. *Drying procedures*
10. *Postprocedure sanitation activities*

- *Add-ons*—A paraffin treatment is a good addition to the manicure and greatly enhances the results.
- *Home care suggestions*—This client should be using a high-quality moisturizing hand lotion several times daily, a cuticle oil twice daily (at least), and a sloughing lotion two to three times weekly.
- *Future appointment recommendations*—A client with severely rough and dry skin needs a sloughing manicure each week, plus a sloughing treatment until her hands have lost their roughness. Then hydrating manicures should be performed until her hands are healed completely. She should have

prescriptive manicures weekly because her hands will have a tendency to return to their rough and dry condition. An exfoliation treatment series will enhance the condition of her skin; return to the hydrating manicures on the completion of the treatments.

This sloughing manicure should take no longer than the usual spa manicure, enabling this upgrade to be almost routine for spa manicurists in some climates. There is a higher charge for this manicure than for the spa manicure. The clients are educated as to the value of the treatment and pointed to the performance of the procedure during the treatment; do not do it in silence or they will not see the value of the increased cost.

Clients like the increased smoothness of their skin after the treatment and will respond to the suggestion routinely, after its introduction.

EXFOLIATING TREATMENT

This treatment is a chemical exfoliation of dead surface cells with AHAs, beta hydroxy acids (BHAs) or enzymatic products. It enhances the natural surface exfoliation to bring healthier, younger looking cells to the surface (see Chapter 10).

An exfoliation treatment is performed as an accompaniment to a manicure or as a separate treatment service. A careful professional with skin care expertise or a technician who is willing to be trained will be interested in doing this service. The home care products are expensive, as is the cost of the treatment, and involves a system of AHA products.

Attention: The only effective way to change the appearance of the skin through chemical exfoliation is in a program. One exfoliation treatment will not show dramatic results toward the resurfacing, though the skin will appear somewhat softer from the effects of the chemicals on the intercellular adhesives. Chemical exfoliation is a slower, more natural process than physical exfoliation and must be performed several times before dramatic results are seen. The process reaches deeper into the layers of the skin and produces more age-defying results. Home care is important to the results in chemical exfoliation and is the secret to the success of the program (no home care means few results).

This program involves a commitment to weekly manicures/treatments with an eye on the result by the client who wishes to have younger, softer hands. Usually the product lines will recommend weekly treatment for 4 to 6 weeks.

In the program, other treatments/manicures are interspersed with the exfoliating treatment, which can be performed as an accompaniment to those manicures, combining a manicure technique with it, making it a manicure, or as a separate treatment. The manicurist does an analysis at every appointment to redefine and identify the services to come.

Exfoliation is hand skin care and has nothing to do with the client's nails though it will exfoliate the cuticles if special attention is paid to them during the procedure.

Client Analysis

These clients will have very dry but probably not rough skin, or systemically dry, sun-damaged, or exposure-damaged skin on their hands, forearms, and elbows. They may have aging skin that needs the dead cells released and the wrinkles reduced.

Exfoliating procedure

The procedure for chemical exfoliation is specific to the product being used to accomplish the process. Typically, the procedure will be surface skin cleansing, skin surface preparation, rinsing, product application, neutralizing/rinsing, moisturization, and application of a sun protectant. If a professional wishes to do this procedure, she must closely follow the directions of the product line she has chosen.

The exfoliation procedure is done immediately after the client is seated. Ideally, the client will have a hydrating manicure following the procedure. SPF lotions are applied after every treatment or manicure and applied daily or more by the client in home care, according to her lifestyle. AHA home care lotions are also a necessity in the home care program for these clients.

Chemical exfoliation manicures are not done on an ongoing basis. Product recommendations should be followed closely, and results should be achieved within four to six treatments. A maintenance schedule is set up after the program.

- *Home care suggestions* — For effective treatments and results, clients should be trained in the exfoliating home care system of the product line and the appropriate products sold to her. These should include a daily regimen of a home care AHA exfoliant product and an emollient lotion, or a high AHA lotion for exfoliation and an emollient lotion. An AHA cuticle treatment and essential oil cuticle treatment are needed, also.

- *Future appointment recommendations* — Maintenance treatments or manicures are prescriptive manicures according to the

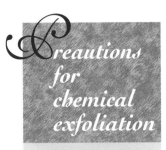

Precautions for chemical exfoliation

Chemical exfoliation has a list of precautions that must be noted and followed (see Chapter 10). A wise spa manicurist will learn them and closely adhere to them. She will also fully understand how the chemicals within the product work and what to do when a problem occurs (see Chapter 10).

spa manicurist's analysis. A bi-annual resumption of the program, such as after wintertime or summer golfing, may be necessary for many clients and can possibly be performed congruent to her seasonal exfoliations for her face.

EMERGENCY MASK

Many product lines contain a mask that can immediately relieve an irritation that manifests during a treatment. If the salon does not have one, find one before using aromatherapy and chemical exfoliation products. A manicurist using these products must learn a procedure for calming and soothing the skin in the case of a rare reaction and keep the products on hand ready for use.

Tepid water will neutralize AHA treatments, and mixtures of 1 tablespoon baking soda in 4 ounces of water will stop the product working immediately. (Many salons require a professional using AHA in exfoliations to keep an application bottle of this mixture handy.)

This is not true for neutralizing aromatherapy reactions. If a client has the rare reaction to aromatherapy, the product should be removed immediately, then the emergency mask applied to calm the skin. The reactions are to the plants and flowers that are the sources for the extracts.

Aromatherapy and chemical exfoliation are safe and effective treatments if the spa professional is fully educated, respects their use, and follows the directions exactly. The results of their use can be dramatic. Clients love the results of aromatherapy products and the feel of exfoliated skin and will return for more treatments, if the manicurist is properly trained, careful, confident, and informed.

AGE-DEFYING TREATMENT PROGRAM

This is a program of prescriptive manicures and treatments. It involves AHA skin treatments, hydrating masks, and home care products, including a hydro-quinone hyper-pigmentation treatment. It has nothing to do with the client's nails except that they are treated during any accompanying manicures. *The same precautions apply for these treatments as for the chemical exfoliation treatments.*

Client Analysis

This client has aging, dehydrated skin, with wrinkles and age spots. Over time, the treatments will take years off the texture and appearance of the client's hands, even lighten the age spots if the client commits to weekly manicures and daily home care. Appropriate home care regimens and prevention with SPF lotions are imperative to the success of these programs.

Age-Defying Procedure

1. The AHA chemical exfoliation treatment is performed, usually six to eight times, once a week, then monthly.

2. A spa or hydrating manicure or hand facial is performed after the treatment, thought without any massage exfoliation.

3. A hydro-quinone product is applied. The client is instructed on its use in home care, according to the instructions of the product line.

4. An SPF 15 or more skin protectant is applied and the client is instructed to use it before every sun exposure.

A spa manicurist who enjoys skin care will be interested in doing this service. The service and retail products are expensive.

- *Home care suggestions* — The hydro-quinone product and SPF lotion must be used daily, indefinitely, as directed for these treatments to succeed. If the SPF lotions are not used routinely, exposure to the sun will cancel any bleaching the hydro-quinone ingredient has done and will darken the age spots. A high-quality hydrating hand lotion is used generously, plus an exfoliating home care system.

- *Future appointment recommendations* — These clients will need ongoing monitoring with prescriptive manicures to maintain beautiful hands. The series should be done twice a year.

NAIL GROWTH PROGRAM

This is not a particular manicure but instead is a program that includes manicures prescribed through analysis of the skin and nails by the spa professional. It involves retail, the matrix massage, weekly appointments, and home care. If a particular manicure is on the menu as a nail growth manicure, it will be the spa manicure or hydrating manicure with the routine addition of a particular massage to the matrix of the nails, using essential oils, and the important use of a nail treatment product (see Chapter 2). These steps are the keys to the success of this program.

The clients see speedy results with this program and love it. It is a great clientele builder: the clients tell their friends or their friends notice their "new hands," and referrals are the result. Any professional who fully develops this clientele will be rewarded both financially and professionally.

The manicures are chosen before each appointment according to the condition of the client's hands and nails. The nail growth manicure can be a staple on the menu of a spa manicurist. However, other hand skin care treatments and manicures can also add two steps, but I suggest the massage and nail treatments not just be assimilated into a manicure or the client will not note their specialness. For instance, a hydrating manicure can add these two steps and the benefits of the nail growth manicure will be included in that manicure, but they should be noted as extras and their performance is an added charge.

Client Analysis

This client will have problems getting her nails to grow beyond the ends of her fingers and many times will have no free edge at all. Many of these clients have *never* had a free edge.

For success of the program the spa manicurist must:

- Assure the client that by working together as partners, she can have beautiful nails in 6 weeks (beautiful, not necessarily long).
- Inform the client that success depends on weekly manicures and her willingness to be a partner in home care.
- Explain to the client the concept of a nail growth program.
- Bring the retail products to the table and inform the client of the place of each in the progress toward success. A 'first needs' list is provided for the products. Example: First week, nail strengthener and aromatherapy lotion; next week, cuticle oil and AHA cuticle solvent, and so on according to analysis.
- Keep her eye on the goals the client wishes to meet and perform the manicures and home care that are needed to meet them.

In a nail growth program, the spa manicurist must inform the client that:

- Her goal is attainable.
- The nail growth program is wonderful, but the nails will not grow out over night.
- Consistent home care with appropriate products will ensure results of the program.
- Nail strengtheners/hardeners dry the cuticles. For this reason, the product should be polished on the nails a bit away from the cuticle.
- A cuticle oil must be massaged into the cuticles at least twice every day, more if the person occupationally or systemically needs it.
- The matrix massage must be performed during application of the oils.

- There may be breakage of the former "bad" free edge, because this will not respond to the treatment well. Many times, breakage of this edge will be a positive result in the long-term plan because the nail appears to respond more quickly after the bad free edge is gone.

- The weekly manicures are necessary to keep the sides of the nails strong as they grow, to "blunt" the nail plate free edge with the proper emery, to give that extra special matrix massage to encourage growth, and to repair any nails that may tear during the process.

- The client is not to attempt to emery her own nails, except for blending a rough area. A non-aggressive emery must be used in this blending.

- Other treatments will be suggested if her skin indicates a need. Beautiful skin is a framework for beautiful nails.

Nail Growth Manicure Procedure

The procedure below is the same as the spa manicure. *Step 4 and step 8 are different from the other manicure procedures.* Other manicures can be the basis for addition of the massage and nail treatment, however, and are recommended prescriptively.

1. *Entrance and seating of the client according to the policy of the salon*
2. *Client analysis*
3. *Remove the polish and shorten/shape the nails/remove obvious dry cuticle*
4. *Hand massage, plus a matrix massage.* The latter massage is specific to the matrix and cuticles of the nail, as described below.
5. *Cuticle treatment/recheck*
6. *Nail bed cleansing/polish prep*
7. *Appointment close procedures*
8. *Nail treatment.* These clients need a nail treatment to treat the conditions of their nails, whether they are normal, peeling, eggshell, or whatever (see Chapter 2). They should be fully instructed on their home care and breaks should be repaired with strip fiberglass.
9. *Polish applied.* Some spa manicurists prefer that these clients not use polish until the treatment stops the peeling.
10. *Drying procedures*
11. *Postprocedure sanitation activities*

- *Home care suggestions* — These clients are taught to perform the matrix massage twice daily with an essential oil cuticle product. A moisturizing lotion and cuticle treatment are in their regimen also. A nail strengthener is essential to this client's success, used according to the recommendation of her spa professional.
- *Future appointment recommendations* — A client on a nail growth program will be a weekly manicure client. Prescriptive manicures are performed weekly, with the accompanying matrix massage and nail treatments. If she stops the care, her nails and skin will return to their former conditions, usually.

Matrix Massage

The hand and arm massages are performed as routine, with one added technique, the matrix massage. In this technique, the matrix area of each finger is massaged. Essential oils are applied to the area, then the professional uses the outer side of her thumb to massage the area. Note that the *soft pad of the thumb is not used*; it is the side of the thumb. The massage area of the professional's massaging thumb is just anterior to the knuckle area, on the side of her thumb.

No massage is performed over three to five times on each finger, and high pressure is not used, because it can be painful. A firm, smooth movement is performed from the tip area of the cuticle side well, toward the posterior, (Fig. 5–10) then around the posterior of the cuticle matrix area, and back down the other side well. (Fig. 5–11) Half of the massaging thumb is on the nail, half is on the cuticle.

Figure 5-10

The Matrix Massage allows for each finger to be massaged.

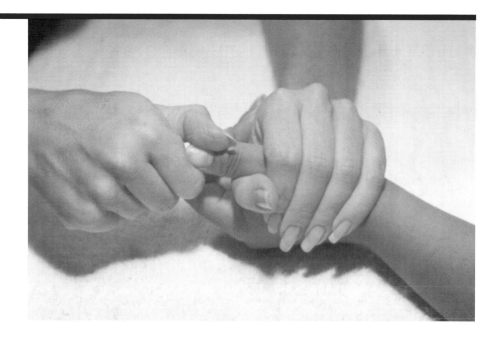

Spa Manicuring for the Salon and Spa

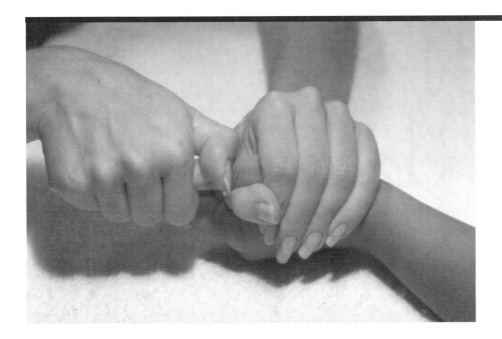

Figure 5-11

The Matrix Massage
is performed around the
posterior of the cuticle
matrix area.

To anchor the massage, arch the index finger that is beside the massaging thumb over the opposite side of the finger that is being massaged. (See pictures.) Now, move smoothly, back across the matrix area and down the other side of the cuticle in a movement similar to the shape of a horseshoe. The professional bends and turns the wrist of her hand that is performing the massage to allow a repetitive swing back and forth. The other hand is merely holding the client's finger from behind.

The professional develops a smooth, arching movement as she becomes proficient with it, bringing a blush of heightened circulation to the area. This enhanced circulation will nourish and stimulate growth in the matrix area, while the oils will moisturize and soften the cuticles and skin around the nail. After the massage, the area is rosy and warm, demonstrating the heightened presence of the blood.

The client is taught the procedure and assigned to use an essential oil that is sold to her as home care. She is encouraged to perform the exercise twice per day, if not more. Those who struggle with getting the time to do it are encouraged to keep it near where they watch TV. ("This is a TV job," they can be told.) Or, they can place it on their bedside table for use at bedtime.

Over the years this procedure has never failed to produce beautiful and strong, natural nails on clients who became my partner in their goal to grow nails. They appoint weekly, do their home care, and their nails grow. Whether it is the oil, the massage, the attention that I give their nails, or their heightened awareness, I cannot tell you—nor do I feel it matters. The fact is, their goals are met and they are happy with their beautiful nails.

NAIL BITER PROGRAM

This manicure program gives extra attention to the cuticles, the nails, and the client as well as dealing with necessary behavior changes. A schedule of appointments (a program) is set up for the client, with retail and home care products and instructions. The specific manicures will vary, according to the analysis of the client's nails and skin.

Mental preparation is important to the success of clients in nail biter programs, as is her spa manicurist's support. She is informed completely of how things will proceed, given assignments, and encouraged and rewarded during each appointment.

Alternative activities are suggested to allow the client to substitute for biting until the habit is overcome. The client may be of any age group, though I suggest only working on those who are mature enough to commit to the manicures and treatments, the required home care, and the suggested alternative activities. This client is a special person and must be treated in a special way. The program works and the clients become permanent residents on the manicurist's client list.

Behavioral Changes

Nail biting is rarely a neurosis or compulsion though it is a very bad habit. Most nail biters can quit, if given a reason (e.g. a wedding) and a way of doing it. This program provides that method.

Most nail biters have already quit when they come in to their manicurist, they just do not know it yet. They may have bit them like crazy on the way to the nail spa, but when they walk through that door, they have quit. Now, it is up to the spa manicurist to maintain their resolve until they come in for their next appointment. Behavioral assignments will help maintain that resolve.

The manicure is important to this process but is actually only the reward. Each week they focus on coming in to have their manicurist say, "You've done so well!" The more important aspect toward the goal is what they do when they are away from the salon, so the manicurist must provide them with *something else to do* to keep them from biting their nails.

First Week Assignments. Amazingly, nail biters may have no idea when they bite their nails. Knowing this is important to their quitting, so the first week, the spa manicurist assigns them this task: "We need you to become aware of when your nails are in or at your mouth so you can tell me next week when you bite your nails." If it will help, ask them to write it down. They are to count how many times each day they catch themselves nibbling and what they are doing at the time.

Send them to the discount store to find a "feeler," a ball, rock, bean bag or whatever. Whenever they feel the need to stick their fingernails in their mouth, they are to begin stroking, squeezing, or grasping that object. It has to be something they can keep with them at all times.

They are taught a home care regimen of matrix massage, AHA cuticle lotions, nail treatments, and hand lotions. For most, just going through the regimen is therapeutic. The regimen is:

- Each morning after their shower they apply oil to their cuticles, then perform the matrix massage. Afterward, they apply the lotion.
- Each evening, they do the same application of the oils, perform the matrix massage, and apply the lotion.

They can do additional treatments if they wish because these routines can many times soften the cuticles, making the nails less tempting, and replace biting. Many persons on this regimen will perform the routine in front of the TV to keep from biting their nails.

Second Week Assignment. Forgiveness for biting one or two nails last week may be important. The list of when they bite is looked over to see if some activities must be redesigned. The object they use as their feeler will be important to these activities. For example, many people chew their nails while they drive, watch TV, or read. The feeler must be used during that time to redirect their activities.

The client has purchased her feeler and the assignment is to use it as much as possible the next week. Most will get through the next week without chewing although their feeler may be starting to show wear. Already, they will be putting their hands to their mouth fewer times than before.

Third Week Assignment. This is a crucial week because they are usually starting to see growth results. Also, they are starting to relax with the thoughts of quitting their habit. The spa manicurist must warn them that this relaxation may cause an unknown nibble. If she is careful to warn them of this possibility, the client will be more likely to cancel the nibble when it happens.

Every week the client must be reminded of the importance of home care and her weekly appointment. Of course, repairs must be performed on broken or damaged free edges to keep them in maximum shape, no matter how pitiful that condition is.

Fourth Week Assignment and on. From now on the routine should be getting toward the positive side of growth and repairs. Remember, no matter how pitiful their nails look to the spa manicurist, *any* free edge is a victory to them. By now, most will be experiencing some free edges as rewards for their efforts. Be certain to shape these tiny free edges carefully because they may be thin. The nail treatments will continue though with a product with less formaldehyde until the free edge is at the length the client likes, then move to a nonformaldehyde product.

The manicurist must reinforce the client's positive feelings weekly, until finally, the nails are beautiful, natural nails with length.

- *Home care suggestions* — These clients will need the spectrum of products: an emollient hand lotion, a cuticle AHA treatment, a cuticle oil, a gentle emery and a nail strengthener.
- *Future appointment recommendations* — Encourage these clients to continue weekly manicures because most nail biters do not care for their nails well. And one little rough edge can start them back on a nail biting spree if they are without the care of their manicurist. Their skin conditions should be addressed because they want to be proud of their "new" hands.

ACRYLIC GROW OFF

Acrylic grow off is a program involving the nail growth manicure, the new basic or spa manicure, and treatment manicures, according to the analysis of the client's skin (see the appropriate related procedures). It is an alternative to soaking off or other removal procedures and is an excellent client retention procedure when a client wishes to remove the acrylics.

Clients will come from other salons to have their acrylics grown off when they hear about the manicurist's ability to gently grow off their acrylics, leaving healthy, strong nails. The procedure involves weekly visits for approximately 2 months, and retail, and leads the client into being a loyal manicure client. Further, this procedure can rid us of having to listen the remark, "Those things ruined my nails."

Nail Grow Off Procedure

The basic procedure for nail grow off is the same as the nail growth manicure with the addition of acrylic retention procedures. Other manicures and treatments may be recommended, according to the condition of the client's skin. The spa manicurist must deal with acrylics that are growing out—aging and crumbling acrylics.

On determining that she wishes to give up her acrylics, the client will be given the options for removal, including the grow off program. If she wishes to go through grow off, the client must be informed thoroughly of the program, as follows:

- This is a commitment to weekly appointments for a particular manicure designed to aid her in this grow off; time is 1 to 2 months.
- Besides the weekly manicures, home care products must be purchased and used regularly as her part in reaching this goal.
- Some breakage is to be expected, and repairs or not are her decision.
- Repairs are designed to continue the nail through the grow off, not to reintroduce acrylics.

Client Analysis

This client is becoming disenchanted with her artificial fingernails. The reasons are myriad; she may have time stresses, money problems, or just be tired of the thoughts of artificial. Whatever the reasons, she will give some indications in her behavior. She may be becoming a chronic complainer about the quality of the work, she may be missing appointments, or she may just seem a bit more grouchy than she was when she first became a client. If the manicurist listens closely, she will be able to define the need to remove them and produce great natural nails during the procedure.

Grow off is not a one-time removal, sending the client off with nasty looking weak nails. The client must commit to weekly appointments until the final result is achieved.

Grow Off Manicure Procedure

1. The client has made the decision to give up her acrylics, for whatever reason, and has decided to grow them off rather than have them removed. Her entrance is routine, as is polish removal. The next step, client analysis, will be specific to removal techniques. She is given the option and description of grow off and has chosen to commit to the program.

2. The posterior borders of the existing acrylics are glued to ensure their retention to the nail bed. In doing so, minor "lifts" are adhered to the nail bed. (Fig. 5–12)

3. The existing free edges of the acrylics are shortened, shaped, and thinned and the natural nail tips glued to the acrylic, when necessary. (Fig. 5–13)

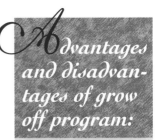

Advantages and disadvantages of grow off program:

Advantages

- The nails are protected in the acrylic-bearing area while the nail behind the acrylics is growing.
- Length can be maintained while the virgin nail is growing.
- The virgin nail is improving in condition while growing.
- The technician can aid the client in maintaining the free edge of any nail where the acrylic accidentally comes off before completion of the grow off.
- The client gradually becomes accustomed to having healthy natural nails and likes them.
- The client can be converted automatically to nail growth program after the acrylics are off.

Disadvantages

- Weekly manicures are a requirement for success.
- Grow off takes time and patience.
- Breakage happens and must be managed with repairs.

Figure 5-12

Glue is placed on the posterior border of acrylic nails to ensure retention to the nail bed.

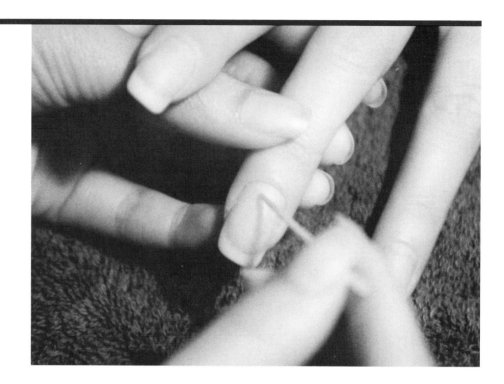

Figure 5-13

Free edges of the acrylics are shortened and shaped.

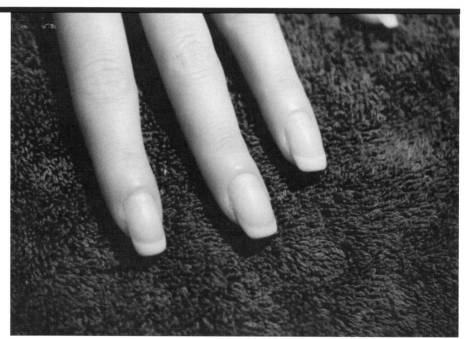

4. The existing acrylic on each nail bed is thinned and smoothed to appear as natural as possible. The stress points are moved to the appropriate areas through filing. **Attention:** Take care to not file or buff on the natural nail.

5. The cuticles are given some attention, matrix massage is performed, and the client is shown how to rub in the oil and perform matrix massage at home.

6. The nail bed is cleansed for application of polish.

7. A nail strengthener/hardener product is applied and the client is properly instructed as to its use in the home care steps. Apply it no more than every 2 to 3 days.

8. Reinforce the home care steps, collect for the appropriate retail, and reappoint.

9. Polish and top coat are applied.

10. A drying procedure is done and the client is released.

The acrylics are shortened, glued and shaped every appointment and the broken nails repaired. If the nail lifts off, leaving exposed nail plate that formerly had acrylic on it, the client should increase her use of the treatment on that area to every other day for a week. After a week, the product is applied daily.

- *Home care suggestions* — Glue, strengthener/hardener product, cuticle oil/lotion, and appropriate skin care are important to the success of this program. The client should be fully informed of the correct use of each product.

- *Future appointment recommendations* — After the first appointment, the skin care needs of the client are addressed in manicures. This client will become a nail growth client as each nail is removed or grown off. Many have never had a free edge without acrylics and will love the feeling of their natural nails. They become a free advertisement of the spa manicurist's expertise and send new clients to the salon. Most will never leave the client list and become sincere advocates of professional nail care. Most will purchase other services and retail from the spa manicurist because they believe in her, as a professional.

Methylmethacrylate Nails

The grow off manicure is ideal for nails that have methylmethacrylate (MMA) product on them. The grow off will protect the nails, hide the damage the MMA has done to the nail plate, and allow the client to maintain a free edge as long as possible. The product should be reduced to *very thin and short*, however, because it will break and lift as its high weight grows to the anterior of the nail bed. A nail strengthener is important to the grow off process with this client.

ACRYLIC MANICURE AND TREATMENT

The manicures or treatments for acrylic wearers are "beautification for their skin," performed between or before fill appointments. They are designed to treat the client's skin care needs, not her acrylics, to treat her to the skin care and pampering that clients with natural nail enjoy. *At these appointments, no work is done on the acrylics unless a repair is absolutely necessary except for a polish being changed or unless it is performed before an acrylic appointment.*

The manicures are chosen through analysis with an eye to extra pampering of these loyal clients while improving the health of their skin. For instance, a client with dry skin will receive the hydrating manicure or hydrating hand facial, or whichever manicure is appropriate to the care of her skin. A client with leathery skin (hyperkeratinized skin) will want the AHA program to soften and brighten her skin.

COMFORT CARE TREATMENTS

This treatment or manicure is for severely chaffed and other very stressed skin, such as those with allergies. Clients with these conditions come to the salon in pain and want relief. The treatment should be performed inside a hydrating manicure and be applied immediately after the massage and before the bagging and paraffin treatment.

The spa manicurist may, through analysis, suggest that this client come in for this treatment two to three times the first week to encourage healing. Home care is important, incorporating cuticle oils and essential oil lotions several times per day. Usually, the healing is apparent by the second week, but if not, she should be referred to a dermatologist.

This treatment should be a calming mask, possibly with chamomile and other calming ingredients. Check with the facial companies because it is available through them already mixed for application. The results are immediate and are teamed later with hydrating masks and treatments in a program to get the client's hands past this condition. The client should be encouraged to continue the manicures and home care as measures of prevention.

Comfort Care Manicure Procedure

1. *Entrance and seating of the client according to the policy of the salon*
2. *Client analysis*
3. *Remove the polish and shorten/shape the nails/remove obvious dry cuticle*
4. *Skin preparation.* The skin prep is performed with makeup remover or gentle sloughing product.
5. *Hand and arm massage/set time in a comfort care mask.* The massage is performed with a high-quality moisturizing lotion, then a comforting mask is applied with a facial brush. The

hands are placed in a plastic bag, then in a thermal hand system (electric mitts) with only medium heat, or warm towels are wrapped around them. They are left 10 to 15 minutes, according to the wishes of the menu designer. The spa manicurist makes certain the client is comfortable for the time she is sitting, and leaves her to relax. After the set time, the mask is removed from the first hand, leaving the second in the plastic.

6. *Cuticle treatment/recheck.* The first hand is treated, then the plastic is removed from the second and it is treated.

7. *Nail bed cleansing/polish prep*

8. *Appointment close procedures*

9. *Polish applied*

10. *Drying procedures*

11. *Postprocedure sanitation activities*

- *Home care suggestions*—These hands need a high-quality moisturizing product that contains hyaluronic acid. This ingredient has very high healing capabilities. The lotion is applied several times daily. An essential oil cuticle treatment is also needed.

- *Future appointment recommendations*—This client may need multiple treatments for the first and second week. Then she is encouraged to continue prescriptive manicures to maintain the health of her skin. Hydrating manicures, hand facials, and sloughing and exfoliating treatments may be needed.

EXTRA TOUCHES

The little extras are what place a spa manicurist ahead of the non-spa manicurist. However, no class on how to do them exists—we have to just pick them up along the way. Below are a few for your consideration:

- *Warm towels*—Clients love that extra touch of warmth in a towel, and the service results are enhanced if the manicurist can add it to her treatments. Of course, the nail spa can purchase a cabbie—they are the ultimate way of heating towels and many spas have them. A crock pot or microwave can also be used.

  The towels must be luxurious because the client will be looking at them for awhile; thin ones do not hold the heat well. If it is to be aromatic, the oil needs to be sprayed on before the folding. Fold the towel in half, length-wise, then roll it tight into a nice neat roll.

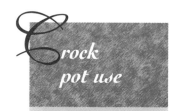

Crock pot use

Cautions in the use of a crock pot for warm towels:

- Wring the towels well. Towels that are too wet can become too hot in a crock pot.

  Take care to not have water in the bottom, or place something there to raise the towels above the water level.

  Do not set the dial on high and leave it there or someone will get burned, or the towels will dry out and stick to the crock pot.

- Turn it off at night to avoid the danger of the towels drying out and catching on fire.

- There is little danger of burning the client as the spa manicurist can sense the heat before it is placed on her—the spa manicurist is the one who gets burned.

To efficiently wet a towel (but not too much) place the rolled end under running warm water, then wring it out as much as possible, until there are no drips. Place several in the cabbie or cock pot.

To use a microwave, place the wet towel (or two) in a closeable plastic bag that is a good fit; the heat will dissipate too quickly in a larger one. Press the air out and close it *almost*, not completely. Now place it in the microwave and heat it for a few seconds. (The professional will have to experiment to find the correct number of seconds because each microwave is different.) Do this either before the client service begins, then close it and place it at your side or in your lap, covered with another towel, or heat it at the time when it is needed, whichever is best for the procedure. Take care not to get them to hot nor too wet. (This takes practice.)

- *Aromatherapy on towels*—Essential oils can be added to wet or dry towels. The most efficient and economical method is to spray or drop a pleasant aromasol oil on the towel before folding and rolling it. Fewer accidents of over-application will happen. Some clients become annoyed when an over-powering amount of oil is used.

- *Crock pots*—Personally, I find the use of crock pots in a nail spa to be a little less spa; however, hot cabbies are expensive, so crock pots are quite often used in that setting until one can be purchased. My suggestion is to place them in the dispensary, out of sight. Then, retrieve the warm towel in a plastic bag, if it is not going to be used immediately, or go to retrieve it at the time of need.

- *Aromatic neck rolls*—The set time for the mitts or a mask should be pleasant and quiet. Aromatic neck rolls that are wonderfully relaxing are available. Some can be heated in the microwave for enhanced treatment and comfort.

Spa manicuring is a new view of client care and is a special mind set for the practitioner. These basic procedures can be the beginning of a highly sophisticated menu for a nail spa, or can be added, one at a time individually by a manicurist who wishes to step up to spa a bit at a time. They are a step above the competition in pampering and results and are developed for professionals who wish to be part of this new concept of client care—spa concept.

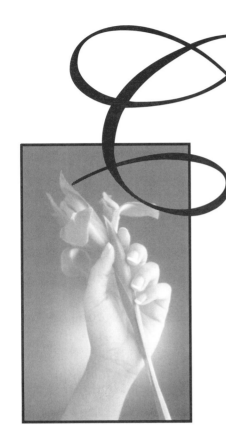

Completing the Picture: Hand Treatments for Estheticians

6

At the end of this chapter, you should be able to:

- Perform an integrated analysis, including the hands.
- Perform hand treatments at the chair side.
- Partner with the spa manicurists in promoting spa treatment.

The skin care procedure taught in esthetics school is a *facial* procedure, not a skin care procedure. Very little is taught on specifics for any other part of the body. When I went to school to become an esthetician I was already a manicurist and, along with new facial skills, I wanted to learn more complex treatments for the hands to use both at the nail care table and at the facial chair. I asked the instructor, "What about skin care for the hands?" Her reply was that during the steaming the esthetician can massage in a lotion on the hands, then put the hands into terry or heat mitts. That was it. I was very disappointed.

After graduating from esthetics school, I used the knowledge I gained to design skin care-based hand treatments for use at the nail table. I also integrated them into my facial routine. How easy are they to use at the facial chair? Basically they are the treatments I described in the spa manicures—just without the nail plate care. Just as the spa manicures, their success depends on one thing: the performance of the analysis step.

ANALYSIS AT THE CHAIR

Estheticians have analysis stressed as the pivotal step within a skin care appointment. It is the secret to client treatment, client education, and home care and the very basis for success in a skin care career. We are taught the mechanics of it, such as where to sit, what to say, and how to recommend treatments and home care. The same must be continued as true for hand skin care analysis at the facial chair. First it must be performed and recommendations and education on the skin care for the hands must be based on it. Second, it must be performed *correctly* or the recommendations will not be accepted. For that reason, I am suggesting that esthetics professionals review Chapters 9 and 10 of this book.

Hand Skin Care Analysis

The hand analysis can be performed before the facial analysis or after it is completed. The main consideration should be that it seems to fit naturally in the facial procedure.

Most of us stand beside the client to do lifestyle and health analysis, then move to the chair behind the client to perform the facial skin analysis. Considering this, many of us will prefer doing the hand analysis before the facial analysis. After the lifestyle and health discussion is completed, it will seem natural to begin the analysis to ask, "Let's see the condition of the skin on your hands first," then reach for her hands to step right into the analysis and make service and home care recommendations for her hands. Then the esthetician moves to her chair to proceed with the facial analysis.

Others of us will prefer doing the facial analysis first and the hands last. After the completed facial analysis, we move to the side of the client and say, "Let's see the condition of the skin on your hands now." Then, we perform a full analysis of the hands, mentioning what is seen to her and go right into recommendations for the hands. (Fig. 6–1)

The analysis should seem as seamless as possible and one of the secrets to this, in adding the hand analysis *after* the facial analysis, unbelievably, is the esthetician's tech chair. To prevent causing a break in the analysis by standing, the esthetician just smoothly rolls the tech chair to the side of the facial chair and reaches for the client's hands. Clients will see this as a continuation of the analysis, then. If the esthetician stands up, it seems to break the analysis and her readiness to listen, into fragments.

I do understand that the size of some rooms or locations of the equipment will not allow this chair movement. If not, as the esthetician stands and moves from the back to the side of the chair she can say to the client, "Let's see the condition of the skin on your hands now." As she moves, she takes the client's hand with one hand, while sliding her other hand from the elbow down to the client's hand, checking the skin. (Fig. 6–2) This will allow some continuous feeling for the analysis. Then, she performs the analysis of the hands, verbally and mechanically.

The analysis should be performed in the same type of movements as the facial analysis. Touch, push, and raise the skin to check for dryness and dehydration. The esthetician should turn the hand over to look at the palms, then point at indications of conditions, such as calluses, generalized keratinization, or dryness. (Fig. 6–3) Recommendations for

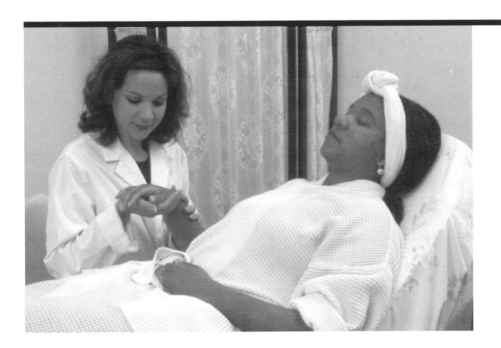

Figure 6-1

A hand analysis is performed and recommendations are made.

Figure 6-2

The esthetician checks the client's skin from elbow to hand.

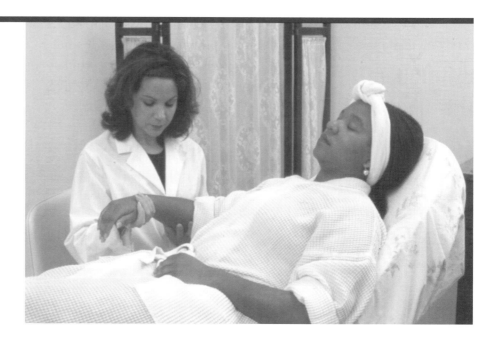

Figure 6-3

The esthetician should examine the client's palms during the hand analysis.

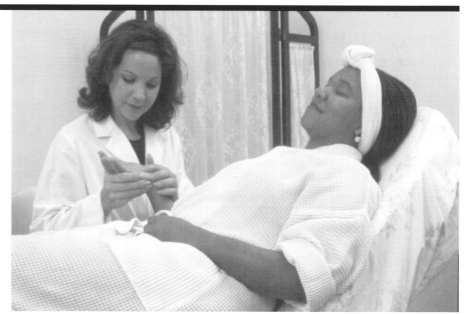

treatments that can be performed during the facial are made, home care products are suggested, and future appointment treatments are mentioned, just as with the face.

The basics are the same as with facial care though there are differences that we need to recognize (see Chapter 9). The same is true here concerning education and home care, however, as with facial skin care—the client must know why a treatment is recommended and her part in extending and continuing the improvement in the skin at home.

The hand treatments can be performed during the service or at separate appointments, according to their complexity or programming.

Most do not add time to a facial, though they still add dollars to the bottom line of the service. They are wonderful upgrades to our care for clients and great book fillers for quick services.

Following are some of the conditions and the treatments recommended. The procedures are outlined later in this chapter.

- *Dry skin* — This client's hands are dry though not rough or chafed. They need hydration therapy. Her hands are usually normal, healthy and hydrated. The cause may be seasonal change or a temporary change in work habits, such as cooking for the holidays or spring cleaning.

- *Systemically dry skin* — This client's skin is *always* dry and will need more aggressive care, such as an alpha hydroxy acid (AHA) series followed by hydrating care and good home care.

- *Rough, dry skin* — This client would need hydration therapy as well as a pretherapy sloughing with a physical exfoliate.

- *Sore, chaffed and dry* — This client's hands need an emergency care mask. This mask soothes and enhances healing while hydrating the skin. She will need several treatments and intensive home care, then will go to weekly hydration therapy treatments for several weeks until her hands are healed and well.

- *Leathery, dry skin* — This client will need an AHA series at weekly visits between her facials (four to six of them), or she can incorporate the treatments into her AHA series for her face. After the treatments she will be referred for weekly hydration manicures.

- *Aging hands* — This client will need an AHA series, as well as hydro-quinone treatments and home care. She will need hydration therapy at every facial treatment, as well as other prescriptive treatments.

- *Paraffin treatments* — Paraffin works well as a treatment enhancer for every treatment *except AHA*. Do not perform a paraffin treatment following an AHA treatment if the AHA percentage is over 30%.

- *Salt glow* — Many spa clients see salt glow treatments as a basic treatment in spas. Many are wonderful physical exfoliators, but the size of the granules must be considered in some conditions. For instance, a client with sore, chaffed skin will not be comfortable with large granules of salt being rubbed across the surface of her skin; small, smoother granules of salt or another physical exfoliate in an essential oil lotion will be just what she needs.

- *Hand reflexology*—A client who would not consider foot reflexology will many times appreciate hand reflexology. The esthetician must be specifically trained in performing it, however. A poor reflexology treatment does not produce results.

These treatments are starter suggestions for an esthetician. Actually, most estheticians have everything they need to develop a number of wonderful and therapeutic hand treatments within their skin care system. All it takes is practice with the analysis and dedication of the purchased products for hand treatments in addition to facials.

Pretreatment Prep

The clients love the lotion-mitt and lotion-paraffin dip treatments that we have done for years. Their hands feel great when they leave and the softness lasts for...all of 3 or 4 hours. How do we make these treatments more therapeutic and longer lasting? With a pretreatment prep. If the skin is more ready to accept the treatments, they will be accepted into the skin and will produce more results.

A pretreatment prep does one or all of the following to enhance the treatment:

1. Removes the oils from the surface of the skin to allow deeper penetration
2. Sloughs the loose, dead cells from the surface of the skin that will interfere with the treatment
3. Combines with the treatment product to enhance the penetration of the ingredients

These products will prepare the skin to accept the product ingredients and allow them to meet their maximum potential for treatment. Pretreatment is a must for the hands, just as it is for the face.

Following are examples of pretreatments that can be used in the recommended services:

1. A good makeup remover will remove the surface oils from the skin ("degrease"), allowing improved penetration of the treatment product.
2. A physical exfoliator, such as a salt glow product, a scrub wash, or a lotion-based exfoliant will remove the dead surface cells, allowing improved penetration of the ingredients.
3. Some products have particular pretreatments that are distinctly designed to pretreat the skin and enhance the penetration of the ingredients. Many AHA systems have these products.

Prescrub

Sanitation is a concern when working with the hands because most contagious illnesses are contracted through touch (see Chapter 13). For that reason, manicurists require their clients to cleanse their hands before sitting down at the table for the service. We do not have that as a possibility for our clients so we must wash the client's hands before the treatment.

The preservice cleansing is performed with a good antimicrobial hand soap or a waterless cleanser after the analysis has been performed and the client has agreed to the treatment. These products are readily available from beauty supply companies. Apply the product generously, massage it into the cuticles and over the hand, and then remove it with a warm, wet towel. After the cleansing and before performing a treatment, the esthetician needs to wash her hands to ensure the removal of all microbes from the treatment area.

After analyzing the hands, the esthetician washes her hands thoroughly to prepare them for the facial service. The hands she had analyzed had not been washed and had contaminated her hands.

HAND TREATMENTS AT THE CHAIR SIDE

Following are the procedures for the treatments listed.

Hydration Therapy

This treatment is the prior-knowledge lotion and mitts treatment with the addition of a pretreatment procedure that will allow the product to penetrate. When you perform the pretreatment, do it with style and elaborate movements. It will appear to be more worth the money that is being charged for the service. A good pretreatment for this treatment would be makeup remover.

1. Prescrub the client's hands with a hand cleanser and towel.
2. Wash your hands.
3. Pretreat the skin with a good makeup remover.
4. Apply a good, aromatic moisturizing lotion and perform a massage. Place the hand in a long plastic bag.
5. Perform steps 1–4 on the second hand.
6. Place the hands in the mitts and allow them to remain there until the service is finished.

7. Remove the mitts and plastic, massage in the remaining lotion.

8. Present the recommended home care products.

- *Home care*—A moisturizing lotion and possibly a cuticle oil should be recommended.

- *Upgrade*—Many spas add paraffin to this treatment. It is applied immediately before the plastic bag. The mitts are put on after the paraffin and plastic bag.

Sloughing for Chafed, Dry Skin

This client needs the dry, dead cells removed form the surface of her skin so that the products can more readily penetrate for healing and moisturizing her damaged skin. Choose a lotion-based slougher, used with elaborate though gentle effleurage movements, or perform a salt glow treatment.

1. Prescrub the hands with a hand cleanser and towel.

2. Wash your hands.

3. Pretreat the skin with a sloughing product.

4. Apply a good, aromatic moisturizing lotion and perform a massage. Place the hand in a long plastic bag.

5. Perform steps 1–4 on the second hand.

6. Place the hands in the mitts and allow them to remain there until the service is finished.

7. Remove the mitts and plastic, massage in the remaining lotion.

8. Present the recommended home care products.

- *Home care*—A home sloughing lotion or scrub and a good moisturizing lotion are needed. A low AHA lotion would be a good product for her to use at home after the healing. She probably will need a cuticle treatment.

- *Upgrade*—Paraffin is often added to this treatment to provide hydration.

Leathery Hands

This client *needs AHAs in a series, weekly*. The treatments take about 20 minutes.

1. Prescrub the hands with a waterless hand cleanser and towel.

2. Wash your hands.

3. Pretreat the skin on both hands with the pretreatment recommended by the system.

4. Apply the AHA treatment as directed by the manufacturer, then put the hands in a plastic bag. Leave it on the hands the recommended time, only. (Usually steps 1–5 can be accomplished during 15-minute facial steam time.)

5. At the end of the treatment time, neutralize according to the recommendations of the manufacturer.

6. Rehydrate the hands with a good lotion.

7. Place the hands in mitts with the heat on low or medium, not high.

8. Remove the mitts after the facial treatment.

- *Home care*—The client *must* use the AHA home care system as recommended by the manufacturer or the treatments will not reach their potential for exfoliation. Full and complete education of the client is necessary. A good moisturizing hand lotion and cuticle treatment are important also.

Aging Hands

The treatment for aging hands is the same as the one for leathery hands with one addition: a skin bleaching or lightening product is applied to the age spots for bleaching. This also is a series of weekly treatments (usually 6–8 weeks). After the AHA treatments, the client is given other prescriptive treatments. The lightening product is applied during these treatments.

- *Home care*—A lightening treatment, an AHA hand lotion, and a SPF 15 sun block product are recommended.

Emergency Care Mask

Most facial systems will have a special mask for sensitive skin or for skin that needs soothing. Incorporate this mask into a hand mask for these sore hands. Use it just as it is recommended to be used on the face. The service should be performed two to three times the first week or two until healing occurs.

- *Home care*—Recommend the client purchase a chamomile lotion for application and removal before bed time for a few days, and a good hydrating lotion for extensive use during the day.

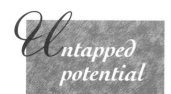

PARTNERING: BUILDING A CLIENTELE QUICKLY

Several of the services at the facial chair are one time services, whereas others should be performed weekly to reach their full potential (aging, leathery hands) for the client. A few may need to be done several times a week initially to achieve healing (hydration for sore, chaffed hands). If the esthetician wishes to perform these skin care services for her clients, that is fine. She appoints the client and does the services. However, many merely want to do the initial upgrade service and the one that will be performed at each facial service the client is scheduled for in the facial chair. This esthetician is more interested in these hand treatments as add-ons rather than as ongoing treatments on a weekly basis. In this situation, she needs a partner to fully meet the needs of the clients and that partner is a spa manicurist.

A partnership between an esthetician and spa manicurist is a situation of mutual benefit. The esthetician analyses the client's skin and does her first treatment, then refers her to the spa manicurist for the multiple follow-up appointments. She discusses the client with the spa manicurist, even introduces them, if possible. She will, however, do the treatment that is due during the next facial as an add-on.

In return for the referral, the spa manicurist will recommend her hand care clients to this esthetician—she is doing skin care of the hands, so the client's facial skin care will come up in the conversation. As a result, each professional will benefit from the referrals of the other professional, and their clientele list will grow quickly. All it takes is a clear understanding of the shared treatments and mutual concern for the clients for a partnership to work well.

Partnering is one of the most untapped clientele builders in salons for all the professionals. A professional who partners with a professional in another department can see their clientele build to "fully booked" in 3 months if they plan together. This partnership between an esthetician and manicurist is especially beneficial for everyone concerned, the esthetician, the spa manicurist, and the client.

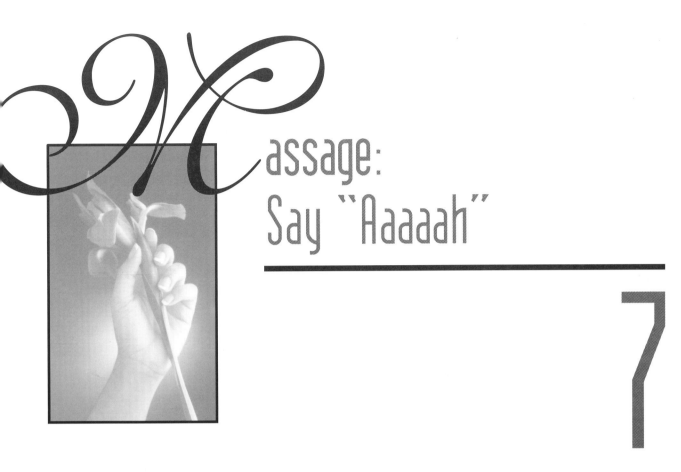

Massage: Say "Aaaaah"

7

OBJECTIVES

At the end of this chapter, you should be able to:

- Define Massage.
- State the requirements for a spa manicurist's massage.
- Describe effleurage, petrissage, tapotement, and vibration in a spa manicurist's massage.
- Describe the physical effects of massage on the systems of the body.
- Describe the psychological effects of massage.
- Name the muscles involved in the hand massage.
- Compare the manicurist's massage to the massotherapist's massage.
- Perform a spa manicurist's massage.
- Hold the hand and fingers in a nontherapeutic manner.
- State the key elements of a spa hand massage.

Massage, a systematic and scientific manipulation of the soft tissue through touch, is an ancient form of healing. The Bible and the Dead Sea Scrolls have many references to healing through touch, often termed the "laying on of hands." Egyptian hieroglyphics show its use as a medical practice in those times, and the Ancient Chinese referred to *Yin* and *Yang* as the essential balance of life and well being, achieved through forms of touch, or massage. The Greek physician and Father of Medicine, Hippocrates, was an advocate of massage, which he defined as *vis medicatrix naturae,* or the body's natural recuperative powers, the "life force."

Massage is a language that speaks directly to the innermost core of our hearts and bodies. It is a very sensitive and sensitizing form of human contact to which humans are very responsive. It seeks and finds causes for pain and stress and replaces them with a heightened feeling of well-being and inner balance. This achievement addresses wellness through *therapeutic* and *stress-relieving* techniques using touch.

Therapeutic massage is "corrective," incorporating a wide range of techniques ranging from deep manipulation of muscles and ligaments to pressing or stroking the skin surface. It can reduce soreness, aid in realigning muscles, and improve performance.

Stress-relieving massage has a different goal. Gentle pressing or stroking of the skin and manipulating the muscles release tension and relax the client. This release leads the client toward a return to a healthful psychological balance within her environment, then helps her to maintain this state of balance.

THE MANICURIST'S MASSAGE

The *relief of stress* is the first focus of massage by manicurists, and we are taught several massage techniques such as effleurage and petrissage to enable us to do just that. However, many of us completely eliminate it or reduce the movements in our routine when we become pressed for time.

Spa requires that we again incorporate massage techniques and purposefully define them. Relaxation is essential to nail spa services. When a client is asked about her spa experience, one of the first things she will mention is the massage…if it was a good one. If not, she will not mention it at all; it was not memorable. As spa manicurists, we want our clients to remember the massage in their treatments as a pivotal experience in their visit, especially because one of the main goals is to relieve tension and stress for our clients. To achieve this, we must analyze our massages, if we do one, then develop one that will meet our clients' goals. Next, we must practice, practice, practice.

The second focus of our massage, as manicurists, is preparation of the skin for our treatments and manicures. The preparation has two phases. First, the epidermis of the skin is softened and warmed through the effects of the massage, enhancing the absorption of ingredients in the lotion. Second, systemic nutrients and moisture are brought to the area via a stimulated and dilated vascular system and the toxins and metabolic products are removed through this renewed vascularization and the movement of the lymph. The open follicles and softened skin will more readily accept the targeted ingredients into the epidermis, and the enhanced nutrients and removal of the toxins will bring an opportunity for a more healthful and rejuvenated dermis. All this is done through the gentle pressing and rubbing movements of our massage.

THE PHYSICAL EFFECTS OF MASSAGE ON THE SYSTEMS OF THE BODY

Far beyond feeling good, massage has an impressive range of therapeutic effects and benefits. It has certain effects on the systems of the body with which manicurists work during a massage.

- *Circulatory system* — Stress and illness can trigger the release of hormones that cause *vasoconstriction*, which is a narrowing of the blood vessels. This narrowing results in reduced circulation of the blood, forcing the heart to work harder, digestion to slow, and breathing to become more rapid and shallow in an attempt to overcome the lower level of oxygen. Massage can help counteract these effects. It can dramatically increase the rate of blood flow; the stimulation of nerve receptors causes improved circulation and increases the levels of oxygen and nutrients through *vasodilation*, which is expansion of the blood vessels.

- *Muscular system* — The direct mechanical effects of rhythmically applied manual pressure and movement can help loosen contracted and shortened muscles and stimulate weak and flaccid muscles. It can maintain the elasticity of tissues through the gentle stretching action it performs to muscles and their surrounding connective tissues. It can speed recovery from fatigue by facilitating the removal of toxins and metabolic waste, allowing more oxygen and nutrients to reach the cells and tissues.

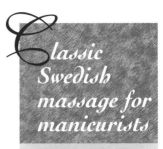

Classic Swedish massage for manicurists

The system of massage called "Swedish Massage" was developed by a Swede, Professor Henry Ling, in the 1800s. His analysis of the many different massage strokes showed the direct physical and psychological benefits of massage and was incorporated into medicine as it was practiced at that time.

Effleurage—A long, sweeping movement that assists the flow of blood and promotes circulation. Its direction is normally toward the heart (from insertion to origin of the muscle) because that is the way the blood flows. It may be deep or superficial in application.

Friction—A circular motion of effleurage that loosens up joints, tendons, and muscles and helps break up deposits and adhesions, small knots of muscle tissue. This movement must be very carefully done by the manicurist, if at all.

Petrissage—A kneading or wringing of the muscles that stimulates the nerve endings, removes congestion and fatigue toxins, promotes flexibility, and assists in contraction of weak muscles.

Tapotement—A light tapping of the muscle that provides an exhilarating and stimulating final movement set in a massage treatment. This stroke increases the blood supply to the surface of the skin, stimulates the nerves, and increases the contraction of the muscle fibers.

continued

continued

Vibration—A light trembling movement of the tissues, performed by placing the hand or fingers on the skin surface and rapidly shaking by trembling, pressing movements. It is stimulating to the nerves and aids circulation.

Some of the Swedish Massage movements are not comfortable nor stress relieving for the manicure client. Wringing is such an example and should not be used in the spa manicure massage routine. A manicurist should always consider the results she wishes to provide the client when designing her massage routine.

- *Skin*—Massage improves the function of the sebaceous (oil) and sudoriferous (sweat) glands. It increases the supply of blood to the skin, thus enhancing the nourishment and moisturization of the tissues. It improves skin tone and promotes vibrant skin. It can enhance the integration of ingredients during skin care treatments.

- *Skeletal system*—Massage relieves aches and stiffness and can increase the range of motion in the joints. It can release muscle tension and free the connective tissue surrounding the joints that may bind them and inhibit flexibility.

- *Nervous system*—The strokes and pressures of massage increase the blood supply to the sensory receptors of the nerves, allowing new nutrients and oxygen to reach the nerve's center. The nervous system becomes more healthful, resulting in alleviation of stress and tension. This promotes a sense of well-being and more healthful and positive responses and reactions to stimuli from the outer world.

THE PSYCHOLOGICAL EFFECTS OF MASSAGE

During massage, the sensory receptors in the skin and muscles awaken to bring the recipient's senses into the present, away from the tension generated by the constant stresses that ordinarily surround her. The resulting release of tension assists in the stimulation of *endorphins*, a hormone in the brain that is one of the body's natural pain relievers. A sense of euphoria can ensue, allowing a temporary "vacation" from day-to-day problems. The immediate result of the relaxation and release of endorphins is the vocalization of "aahs" and relaxing sighs and deep breathing. All massage professionals see these responses as signs the clients are receiving the special psychological effects that massage produces along with the physical effects.

Massage also benefits the professional who provides the massage. It is an experience in giving that quiets the provider's mind and redirects her attention from herself to others. Research shows that blood pressure is lowered, also.

The message is that some clients see massage as an important form of "drugless therapy" and view it as an important component of their health maintenance and wellness plan. They purposefully seek out a professional who performs the best massage during their services, whether the services are skin care, manicure, pedicure, or body work.

THE PHYSIOLOGY OF HAND AND ARM MASSAGE

Our hands are complex instruments. Examine your own closely. The wonders of their structure, sensitivity, and strength are surpassed only by their marvelous ability to perform intricate and incredible tasks. This intricate design and the integral and related actions of hands and arms are basic to performing a massage. The effective professional strokes, kneads, pushes, pinches, and feathers, all in the same set of touches. At the same time, she guides the pressure of her fingers to ensure gentleness with firmness. She also senses soreness, pain, knots, and tension so that no harm will be done. All this is through wondrous hands and fingers!

While she is providing a massage for a client in a pleasant and soothing manner, a manicurist is aware of the physiology of the musculature that she is working with. She knows where they are located, their *origin* (the fixed portion of a muscle, attached to the skeleton) and their *insertion* (the moveable end of the muscle), and becomes aware of the results of the action of its *belly* (body of the muscle). She knows the activity each muscle will control and the particular movement of the body it will allow.

The pressure of a massage moves the toxins and wastes from the muscles toward elimination, allowing increased vascularization of the areas and enhancing nutrition for the muscles and skin.

THE MUSCLES IN THE HAND MASSAGE

The muscles routinely involved in the hand massage activities of a manicurist are the muscles of the forearm, the muscles of the hand, and their accompanying tendons. These muscles are:

1. The *pronators* (pro-**nay**-tors) turn the thumb and the hand inward toward the body so the palm faces backward or down. It moves the distal end of the ulna across the radius. This is the most comfortable and usual position of the forearm and hand.

2. The *supinators* (**sue**-pi-nay-tors) turn the hand outward with the thumb away from the body, and the palm facing forward or upward. (The arm is in the anatomic position.) The radius and ulna are parallel.

3. The *flexors* (**fleks**-ors) bend the wrist upward, drawing the hand up, and close the fingers toward forearm and palm.

4. The *extensors* (eck-**sten**-sors) straighten the wrist, hand, and fingers to form a straight line.

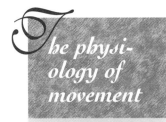

The physiology of movement

Body movement occurs when muscles contract or are shortened across joints. Each muscle is attached to bone or other connective tissue structures at two points or more. One is the origin, the immovable or least movable, and is attached to the less movable bone. The insertion, the movable part of the muscle, is attached to the bone to be moved. When the muscle contracts, the insertion moves toward the origin, moving the bone. Usually the origin is closest to the heart.

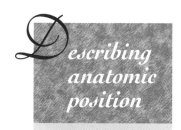
The many small muscles of the hands enable flexibility, strength, and finite intricacy in the movements of the hands. Many of the tasks of these small muscles are performed through control from afar by muscles in our arms, much like the control of puppets. The tendons attaching these larger muscles to the smaller muscles of the hands allow the larger muscles of the forearms to control these movements in the hands and wrists. What an innovative and marvelous design! Think about this: If this marvelous system were not designed in this manner, the constant movement of the muscles in our hands would cause them to grow large — too large for the finite movements we need to maintain our life.

MANICURISTS' MASSAGE VERSUS MASSOTHERAPISTS' MASSAGE

The manicurist's massage is a "feel good" massage, with beautification of the skin an additional benefit. It is not intended to have any deep muscle therapeutic movements, we are not trained for it nor is that our purpose in a nail spa. The spa manicurist's massage should not have any deep muscle movements.

The difference in the focus of the massage therapist's and the manicurist's massages requires that manicurists hold their fingers and hands differently than massotherapists during the massage. The massage therapist's hands and thumbs are held in a controlled, strong, "inner curve" stance. (Fig. 7–1) This professional's fingers and hands are targeting specific muscles for defined reasons and performing movements for defined manipulations. The hold on the hands and arms is firm and controlling, when properly done. Conversely, the manicurist's hands are held in a more gentle stance. It might be considered an "outer curved" stance. (Fig. 7–2) The gentle strokes are not targeted to specific muscles and do not perform defined muscle manipulations. The thumbs and fingers are expanded, instead of contracted inward. The pressure should be more from the inner side of the knuckles of the fingers and the palms of the hands than from the fingertips. (The exception to this is reflexology, which is discussed in Chapter 8.)

The spa manicurist's thumbs and fingertips are not pressed against the skin and muscles of the client; instead, her inner *knuckles* exert the pressure on the skin and muscles. Practice removing "control" from the tip of the thumb and fingers, exerting the pressure at the first knuckles, the fingers and with the palm of the hand. (Figs. 7–3a and b) When holding the client's wrist, place pressure only on the knuckles, allowing the fingertips to relax. Pressure exerted against the client will not be strong and specific, and you will see a more relaxed client.

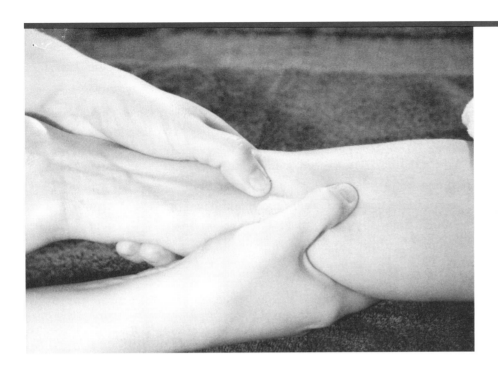

Figure 7-1

The massage therapist's hands use finger pads in massage techniques.

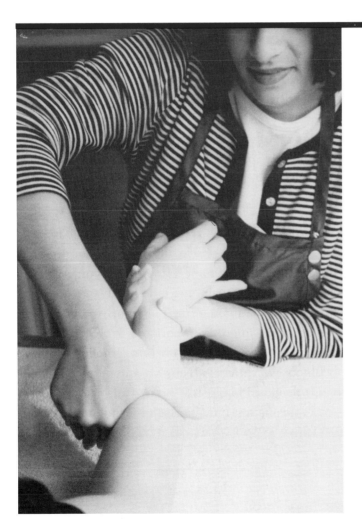

Figure 7-2

The manicurist exerts pressure by using the inside of the knuckles, not pads, of fingers.

Figure 7-3a

Incorrect position—stronger
grip can hurt client.

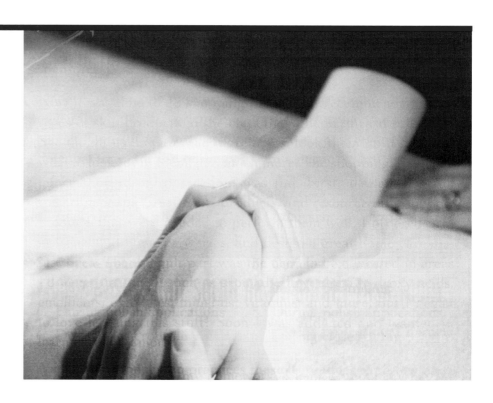

Figure 7-3b

Correct—pressure is exerted
by the inside of the knuckles.

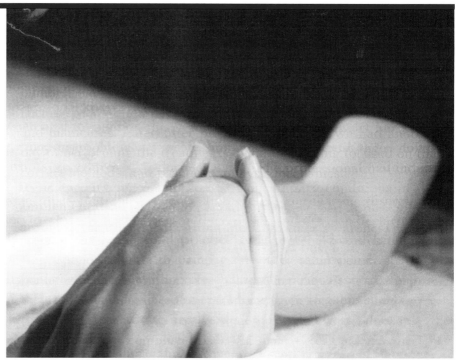

This described massage stance *can* be done while wearing artificial fingernails. The massage therapist's *cannot* be done with fingernails
beyond the pad of the fingers. The pressure of the manicurist is over a
general area, whereas, the massage therapist's is targeted to a specific
muscle or group of muscles.

The manicurist who wishes to perform the best and most relaxing massage must practice the firm, though gentle, manicurists' hand stance. It can successfully provide a stress-relieving, feel good massage, while warming the skin and encouraging the absorption of the treatment products. All this can be done without going beyond our training and capabilities and still meet our objectives. If a client requests a massage requiring more expertise in therapeutic massage, she must be referred to a trained, certified massage therapist.

SPA MANICURE MASSAGE PROCEDURES

A professional massage procedure is defined by the personality and degree of thoughtfulness of the provider. A professional who is focused on her own schedule and her own rewards will reflect this in the development and execution of her massage procedure. The movements may be jerky and quick, even rough, inadequate massage lotions/oils may be used, resulting in a "drag" on the client's skin, and the manicurist may even talk during the manipulations, a "no-no" in spa manicuring. The client will not enjoy this important aspect of the manicure as much as she should.

Massage for the serious manicurist is a personal thing. She takes what she has learned in school, then develops her own regimen. There are petrissage, effleurage, reflexology techniques, and more. Any movement is correct, as long as the spa manicurist is trained and it is not uncomfortable to the client.

However, we hope to produce more than relaxation with the massage in a spa-type manicure. We want our stress-relieving massage to enhance the results of our skin and nail care service as well and, for that reason, I recommend adding several movements to a personal massage pattern that will:

1. Stimulate the flow of blood to the hands and the tips of the fingers
2. Stimulate the presence of the natural moisturizers from the lower layers of the epidermis
3. Massage and slough the elbow, when necessary
4. "Drain" the arm

I emphasize here they are added; the rest of the massage is according to *the manicurist's own design.*

The caring and client-focused spa manicurist's massage will be slow, gentle, and relaxing. For many of us, this takes concerted effort! We have to slow down to give a truly spa massage. We have to take deep breaths, use personal relaxation techniques, and even count the movements to be certain we include them all. It is worth it for the client in the end!

One characteristic of a spa manicure massage is that all movements are connected. The hands are never taken completely away from the hand or arm; there is always a connecting movement. The manicurist develops an even, firm group of movements. The quality of the movements is in the smooth, even pressure, not in the high number of repetitions. Three right hand and left hand movements, slowly and evenly are better than ten, jerky, high-pressure movements. The palm massage movement (the butterfly movement) is performed between each of the other massage movements through few repetitions.

One of the manicurist's palms is always held against the client while the other may be moving to the next area. For example, when moving from the palm to the fingers, one palm is against the side of the hand stabilizing it while the other is moving into position on the first finger.

The massage is initiated by warming a generous portion of lotion between the manicurist's palms or retrieving it from a manicure heater, then applying it slowly over the entire hand. An initial wrist relaxation movement should be executed before moving to the palm.

Palm Massage

This movement is a type of effleurage over the palm and the positioning of the manicurist is important to the effectiveness of this movement. The manicurist's elbows are on her side of the table, about one-third the distance toward the client and a maximum of 3 to 4 inches apart.

I take the client's hand in mine and place her elbow at approximately the center of the table or slightly toward her side of it. I guide the elbow to that position by taking her hand in my left hand, placing my other hand gently on the inside of her elbow, and pulling it forward. (Fig. 7–4)

Palm Massage Routine. This movement is a butterfly movement of the thumbs on the palm of the hand. Hold the hand with the left hand; the holding pressure should be apparent only on the inside of the first knuckle of each of the manicurist's fingers. The pressure should be even and gentle, in a form of a "c," from the finger, around the hand and down the thumb. (Fig. 7–5) Never allow the fingertips or thumb of the holding hand to fold in and exert pressure.

The other hand is also holding the hand, with the thumb at the base of the "lifeline" on the palm. Most of the pressure is from the knuckle back to the base of the thumb. Do not allow the thumb tip to apply as much pressure as the knuckle. (Do not fold it in to apply pressure.) (Fig. 7–6)

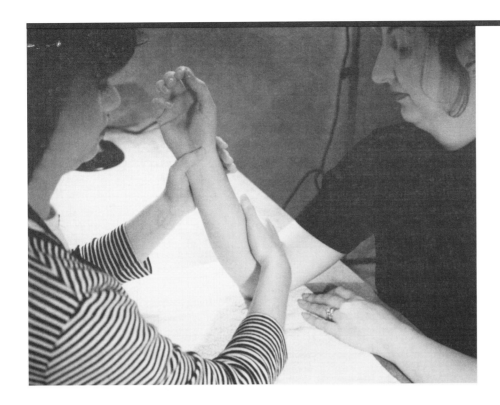

Figure 7-4

The client's arm is pulled forward with gentle guidance by the spa manicurist.

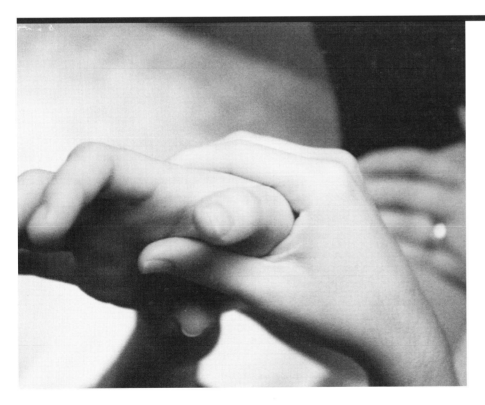

Figure 7-5

The manicurist's hand forms a "c" around the client's hand.

Slide the thumb across the palm of the hand, upward toward the opposite side of the palm, allowing pressure across the entire inner palm with the inner part of your thumb and its base. Come across the top of the palm, just below the base of the fingers, and down the other side of the palm. Return to the lifeline area of the thumb. The hand will be stabilized in place now with that hand.

Slide the left thumb to the base of the lifeline area at the heel of the palm. Slide it up, as with the other hand (on the other side of the hand), across the hand below the fingers, down the side and back to the lifeline area.

The full palm is massaged with this movement, first with one thumb by the spa manicurist, then the other, relaxing the hand and bringing the blood to the area along with heat and nutrients to the skin.

Finger Massage

This movement is designed to relax the fingers and bring abundant circulation to the fingertips and as a result, stimulate the removal of toxins. This initial push movement is light, while the pull toward the fingertips is more firm.

Finger Massage Procedure. After the butterfly movement, reapply ample lotion. Take the client's hand with your nondominant hand,

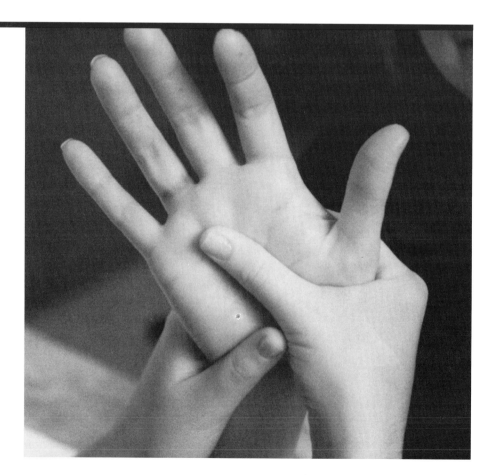

Figure 7-6

Only one thumb is moving on the client's hand at a time.

holding it at the wrist-hand junction with the thumb on top, the fingers underneath as previously described—gently, with no pressure on your finger and thumb tips.

With your other hand, *palm up,* place your thumb on one side of the fingertip, your index finger, crooked, on the other side of the fingertip. (Fig. 7–7) Gently push them to the base of the finger. (Fig. 7–8) Now, roll your thumb up and over the top of the finger, back to underneath the finger. Slide the thumb and index finger, with the rotation being done by the rotation of your wrist, like turning a door knob. (Fig. 7–9) The thumb will now be beneath the finger, on the bottom side, and the index finger will be arched over the top of the finger. Pull your thumb and index finger toward the nail tip while *gently* squeezing them on the finger. (Fig. 7–10) The thumb is against the bottom of the finger. Lightly pinch the tip of the finger as you slide along it, (Fig. 7–11) then turn over the finger along the cuticles and matrix and restart the massage movement (the door knob is being turned the other direction.) (Fig. 7–12) Again, speed of movement is not the issue here; even, smooth pressure and firmness produce a deep, stimulating massage and "pull" the blood toward the fingertip. I usually do three to five on each finger. After you have performed the movement on each finger, you turn the client's hand so you can again massage the palm in the method described above.

Along with these movements, I turn the hand and massage the back in a circular movement with my palm (some persons feel pain when the fingers are used), add any other movements that I see are important to the client, and do a closing routine. Between other movements,

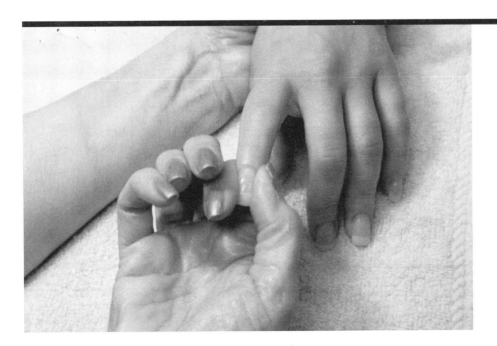

Figure 7-7

Finger stance—grip sides of fingertip at the cuticle.

Figure 7-8

Push gently to base
of finger.

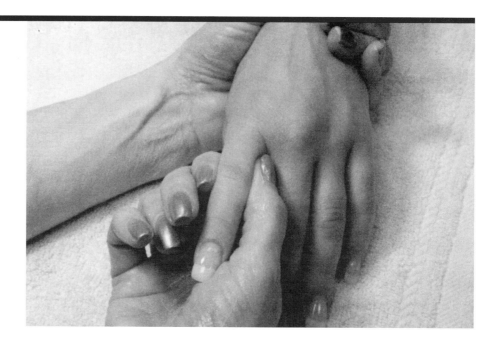

Figure 7-9

Rotate fingers counter-
clockwise, so thumb comes
over the top of finger.

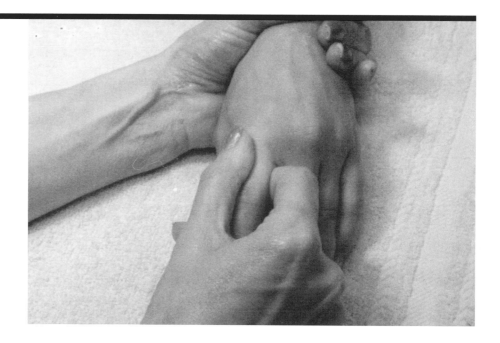

I return to the palm and perform a short palm butterfly to keep the
blood flowing and the heat up.

The number of different movements used in a massage is not as important as the relaxation of the client.

After completing the hand massage, the spa manicurist wraps the hand
to enhance the spa effect, according to the dictates of the manicure
procedure, then moves on to the arm.

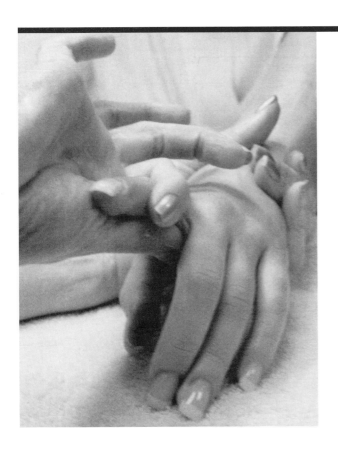

Figure 7-10

Exert gentle pressure against client's finger while pulling toward nail tip.

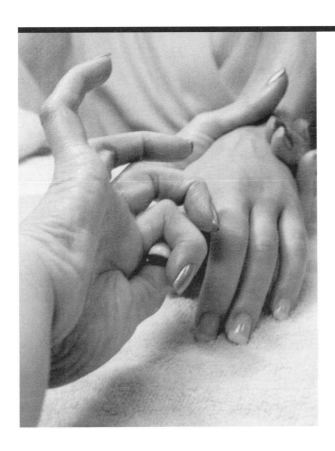

Figure 7-11

Thumb is now flat under finger and index finger is arched over the top.

Figure 7-12

Reverse the direction to start the massage movement.

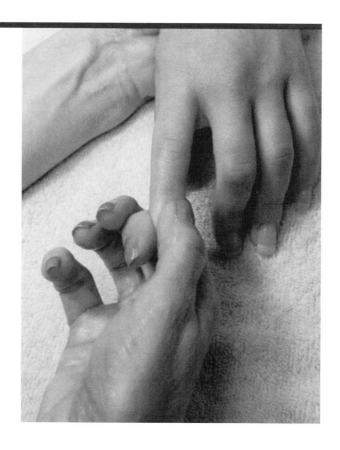

Arm Massage

The arm movements of the massage are the most neglected by manicurists, despite their necessity for the manipulative and enhanced removal of the toxins, the relaxation of the client, and the enhanced nutrition of the hand. The initial motion of the arm massage is an especially important movement for the effectiveness of the massage because it promotes the removal of the toxins after the prior hand massage.

Arm Massage Procedure. Apply more lotion from one hand while gently stabilizing the wrist with the other. (Fig. 7–13) I suggest that you do not massage the arm with both hands at once as many of us were taught in school. If you do so in the firm, even pressure that is appropriate to a good massage, the client may be pushed back and forth in a "bouncing" motion. Instead, hold the wrist as described earlier and massage with the other hand. She can relax, knowing she will not be knocked off her chair; she is in your capable and gentle hands.

The hold is the gentle, fingertipless hold, as described previously. (Fig. 7–14) Hold the wrist of the arm with this no-fingertips hold and use the base of your palm and the base of your thumb of the other hand in a firm, even movement to move the lotion *up* the arm toward the elbow in a sliding movement. (I prefer a relaxed encasement of the arm in a "c" configuration of the thumb and fingers for the movement. No tight fin-

Spa Manicuring for the Salon and Spa

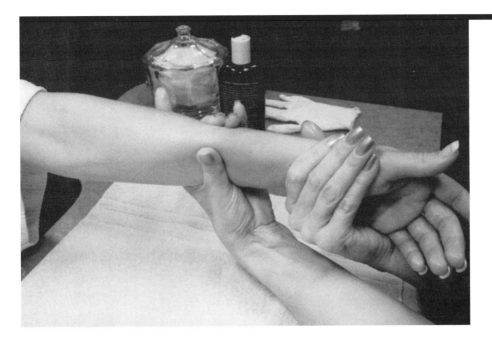

Figure 7-13

Be sure not to grip your client's arm tightly with your fingers.

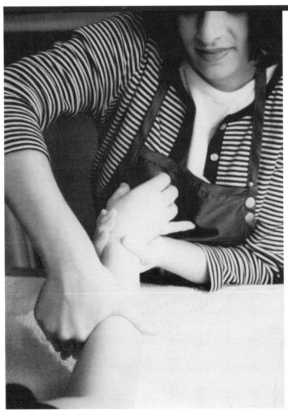

Figure 7-14

Use a firm, even movement to slide the lotion up the client's arm.

gertips, of course.) Massage therapists describe the function of this movement as "draining" the arm or moving components of the blood and lymphatic system toward the heart. After each movement, turn to the wrist area with a lighter touch (*firm* up, *light* down). This movement will move the toxins released from the hand and arm away from the area. At this time, some spa manicurists like to add a gentle, circular, surface movement on the surface of the skin from above the wrist toward the top of the lower arm. (Fig. 7–15) If so, perform it after the draining movement. Perform several movements up the arm. Now, change hands to massage the other side of the arm in the same manner.

If you sense areas that feel like a knot in the client's muscle, pressure should be lightened, but the area massaged directly. (Take care not to hurt the client.) The area can be left after a light massage then remassaged gently several times—this will usually relax or eliminate the "knot."

Elbow Massage

Continue to hold the hand at the wrist. Apply lotion to the palm of your hand and massage the elbow with the palm of your hand. (Fig. 7–16) (Many people have sensitive elbows and do not like to have their "crazy bone" touched; using your palm will alleviate this possibility.) You may want to use a tiny amount of sloughing lotion with the chosen lotion to give your elbow massage a sloughing quality. (Sometimes only sloughing lotion is used.) Again, do not be tempted to use many quick movements; a few and even pressure is much better.

Ending

After the elbow, a gentle "pull" movement down the arm will stimulate the client's circulation. Hold the arm with one hand as described before, circle the arm with your lotioned fingers and thumb in a "c" and with an even and firm but gentle squeeze, pull the lotion toward her hands. (Do not squeeze hard, just firmly.) You may want to use

Figure 7-15

Use a gentle slide to return to wrist.

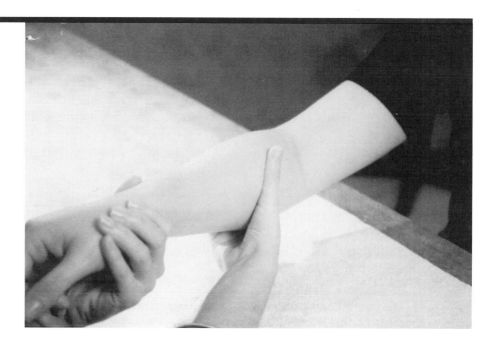

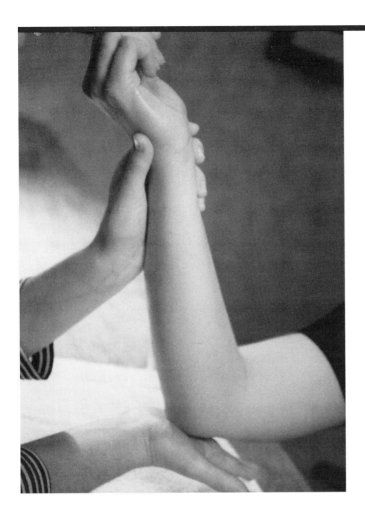

Figure 7-16

Proper hold to begin
elbow massage.

this movement to add lotion to the skin surface of the arm to supply
additional moisturizing for penetration during the set time.

Reapply plenty of lotion to the client's hands, massage her palms and
fingers in a closing movement of your choice, and apply cuticle soften-
er to the cuticles. Then, wrap her hand and arm as the manicure or
treatment requires and move on to the other arm. Warmed towels are
wonderful, but not a requirement. (It is best to use dry towels; wet
towels will dry out the surface of the skin and/or cause a chill during
the cooling off period.) Spa manicures usually include encasement of
the arm in a plastic tube bag, possibly even paraffin to enhance the spa
quality of the procedure, see Chapter 5).

Be certain to use enough lotion when massaging. If you are using moisturizing lotions for massages, this may require a lot of lotion, which
may have to be added several times.

Massage is where our old "hot oil" lotion heater can come back into
use. For an optimal massage with enhanced results, place the massage

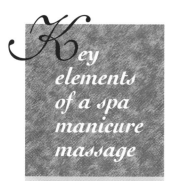

Key elements of a spa manicure massage

• When massaging, be certain to use plenty of lotion.

• The caring and client-oriented professional's massage will be slow, gentle, and relaxing.

• All movements are connected. The hands are never fully released from the hands or arm.

• The palm massage is a continual, butterfly-like movement.

• The palm is massaged between all other massage movements on the hands.

• The wrist is held in a gentle, fingertipless hold.

• The pressure of a comfortable massage is usually from the insertion toward the origin, or toward the heart.

• The hand massage has two focuses: stress relief and enhancement of the absorption of the product.

lotion in the heater and apply and reapply from there, using a spatula. It will not really warm in the beginning because it was not filled until after analysis. After a few minutes, it will be very warm and soothing. (Many spa manicurists warm it in a microwave ever so slightly—a few seconds is enough—to give it that little boost for the start.) The clients love it!

After the massage, the client's hands and fingers feel warm, the color of the skin is more rosy and healthy in appearance, and the cuticles and matrix area of the fingers are reddened from vascularization. The muscles will feel relaxed, though invigorated. The clients note these pleasant and soothing effects of the massage, and many will return to the professional just because of the well-performed massage.

INCORPORATING MASSAGE

If massage is new to you, do not be concerned; with practice on your newly designed massage techniques, you will soon hear those "aaaaahs." However, before working on paying clients, practice your new technique on any one who will lend you their hands. Family, friends, fellow professionals, and your boss will love to take time out to allow you to practice. They will be back for more! They will love the stress relief you provide and will be saying "Aaaaaahhh!" Just as important, you will enjoy performing such an immediately rewarding service.

Hand and arm massage must take on a whole new meaning to a nail technician who wishes to become a spa manicurist. The dedicated spa professional quickly realized that the results of every spa manicure service may depend on the skill and completeness of the professional's massage.

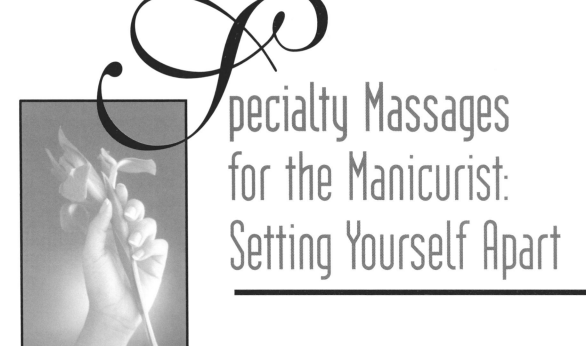

Specialty Massages for the Manicurist: Setting Yourself Apart

8

OBJECTIVES

At the end of this chapter, you should be able to:

- Define aromatherapy.
- State how essential oils perform.
- Define reflexology.
- Seek out a credible reflexology course.
- Compare foot reflexology and hand reflexology.
- Describe how reflexology is performed.

Spa manicurists are one step or more ahead of others in their profession, and the clients expect their care to be distinctive. One of the ways a spa manicurist can distinguish herself is through specialty massage techniques. These techniques take education and practice. Among them are aromatherapy and reflexology massage techniques.

AROMATHERAPY MASSAGE

Essential oils have been used since antiquity in the art and science of healing and to soothe the body, mind, and spirit. These precious oils are highly concentrated, nonoily, volatile extracts distilled from the aromatic roots, stalks, flowers, leaves, or fruit of plants. Each oil contains its own unique beneficial properties, which are used in aromatherapy. They contain vitamins, minerals, and natural antiseptics and have hormone-like qualities that are recognized by the aromatherapy specialist. (Fig. 8–1)

Aromatherapy is a term coined by Professor Gattefosse, a French scientist, for defining the use of essential oils as the "therapeutic use of odoriferous substances obtained from flowers, plants and aromatic shrubs, through inhalation and application to the skin." As spa manicurists, we use them as treatment oils and in lotions for our massage and as enhancements for relaxation through their aromas. The terms aromatherapy, aromatherapy oils, aromatic oils, and essential oils are used in referring to this science and its substances.

Figure 8-1

Aromatherapy massage uses essential oils.

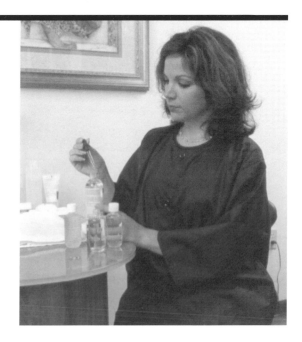

Essential oils work in two distinct and different ways but can accomplish both in the same service. They work through their unique aromas affecting the sense of smell and by absorption through the skin. These properties of the oils are used in manicures called aromatherapy manicures, in pedicures called aromatherapy pedicures, and in massages called aromatherapy massages, in which their aromas are used in tandem with massage. This effective combination can invigorate a client as well as promote her healthful relaxation. These treatments are much sought after in nail spas.

Aromatherapy has moved into the mainstream within the last 10 years. It is now being offered in upscale salons and spas throughout the world in wonderful therapeutic and de-stressing treatments. These treatments are simple to add to existing menus and the clients respond to their therapeutic attributes immediately. The clients are easily convinced by their inviting aromas to add their benefits to their home care.

THE PHYSIOLOGY OF AROMATHERAPY

When clients think of aromatherapy, they think of the fragrances emitted by the essential oils. These scents are carried, via the nostrils, directly to the limbic system of the brain. This system is the center for directing hunger, thirst, memory, and heart rate and is associated with various emotions and feelings, such as anger, fear, sexual arousal, pleasure, and sadness. It also gauges the dissemination of hormones and the sex drive. It is thought that the individual scents direct different subtle responses through this limbic center.

The choice of essential oils for use within the massage can be complicated for the novice and warrants cautions. For example, essential oils of rosemary should not be used on persons with high blood pressure. To help with this problem, several companies have prepared blends of oils safe for use by manicurists and facialists in aromatherapy massages, with specific directions for safe use. For instance, *Yin* and *Yang* blends of oils are available for use in massage lotions. A Yin Oil is a relaxing blend of natural essential oils for clients who are hyper or stressed; a Yang Oil is an energizing blend of natural essential oils for clients who are tired and lack energy. These oils can be chosen by the manicurist to promote the Yin or Yang attributes within the client during the massage.

Prepared and blended oils are available labeled with descriptive words, such as tranquility, invigoration, energizing, and relaxation, among others and would be a blend of oils for achieving these states of being.

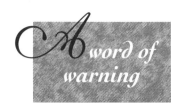

A word of warning

Aromatherapy is a delightful enhancement to the manicurist's expertise, but requires study, followed by safe and skillful application of the knowledge gained. Essential oils are very powerful. Therefore, unless a professional is prepared to study the intricate attributes of the volatile oils, she should stick to the prepared oils and consider their application only as specifically directed.

Essential oils are considered medicines in Europe because of the potential changes they may foster in the person to whom they are directed. They are dispensed by doctors and pharmacists and used only by experienced, professional qualified practitioners. Therefore, if a nail spa incorporates them into their professional practices of manicuring, the oils should be treated with the respect that something unknown deserves.

The names and aromas of these oils will spark the interest of the client and provide aromatic support for the manicures.

Some manicurists have studied aromatherapy and chosen a menu of oils for potential use in their massage lotion. They choose the oils possibly even blending them into interesting aromatic mixtures for use in the massage, or they allow their client the choice, explaining to them the attributes of the oils available to them.

Essential oils do not usually mix with water. Therefore, specially blended water-soluble essential oils or aromasols must be used in aromatherapy compresses (warm, wet towels infused with oils). These are pure essential oils blended into three to four parts emulsifier.

If you wish to learn more about aromatherapy, an abundance of information is available on the subject, some written especially for manicurists. The facial, nail, and massage professional trade magazines often have articles on aromatherapy. Call them and ask for reprints, or if you are a subscriber to one, look in their article index in their December issues for articles that were written on the subject that year. You may already have them in your stacks of trade magazines.

If your interest continues, check out books by experts in the field on the subject. Many are available through Milady Publishing, at large book stores, and at your library. If your library has none, they can obtain them on interlibrary loan if you have the name of the book and author. The publisher's name helps.

Courses are often listed in the books written on the subject. There may also be listings of available classes in the Calendar of Classes in the back of trade magazines. Courses on aromatherapy are available for interested practitioners and a professional who wishes to go beyond the use of the premixed blends and the all-around oils, such as lavender, chamomile and eucalyptus, *should* seek out this training. (Figs. 8–2a, b, c)

For our use, aromatherapy is a spa technique that provides immediate results, such as the general relaxation and rejuvenation effects for the client and the softening and healing effects for the skin. The oils can be added to our services to produce their specific effects and are used as ingredients in our therapy products. The results of the services are enhanced and clients appreciate the use of this skill in their services. It must be stressed again, however, that a professional must study the use of essential oils to become aware of their mixing nuances and many cautions *before* beginning to use them in any complexity.

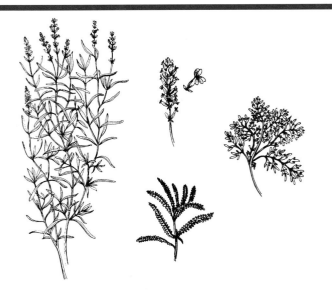

Figure 8-2a

Lavender.

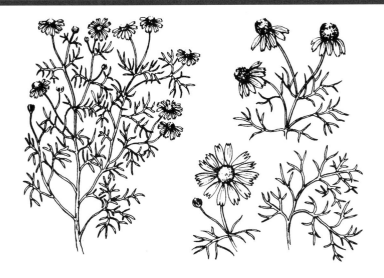

Figure 8-2b

Chamomile.

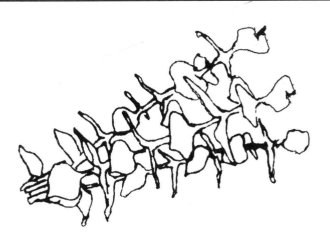

Figure 8-2c

Eucalyptus.

REFLEXOLOGY

Generally, the massage techniques taught in the beauty schools are Swedish massage techniques (see Chapter 7). However, practicing manicurists are becoming interested in learning other techniques and incorporating them into their services. Reflexology is one of those techniques.

Reflexology is based on an ancient *pressure point therapy* theory, a form of thumb or finger compression applied to specific points on the hands and feet. In this massage, pressure is applied with the tip of the thumb or index finger, then it is slowly inched over the area in a steady and rhythmic movement termed walking.

Reflexology is an ancient form of Chinese medicine rediscovered in China by Dr. William Fitzgerald in 1913 and introduced to America through his teachings. It refers to a type of pressure point massage based on *zone therapy* that releases *energy blockages* through the manipulation of specific pressure or energy points on the body. Zone therapy maintains that the body can be divided into ten zones, five on each side of a middle, vertical line on the body, represented by the spinal column. Theoretically, all five zones on the corresponding side of the body are "reflected" in each hand and foot. (Figs. 8–3 and 8–4)

The theory of reflexology is that any tenderness felt in an area of the foot or hand during the massage is said to be reflecting an imbalance from the corresponding body area, not to pressure in the foot or hand. Also, if one has a pain in a certain area of the body, reflexology massage may assist in discovering which organ is responsible for the pain or sensitivity; massage of that area of the hands and feet will reflect positive energy to the area or organ. This positive energy is said to enhance the natural healing process and foster a feeling of well-being and relaxation. Pressure point massage is said to aid in prevention of the development of disease. It is not represented as a healing procedure, however.

In this theory, all organs situated on the corresponding side of the body will be sensitive to massage in a specified area of the foot or hand. For example, the eyes, ears, and sinuses on the right side of the head are reflected to the areas on and around the toes or fingers of the right hand and foot, whereas the spine is vertically referred from the inner edge of both feet or hands because of its presence in both sides of the body. The colon is on the lower soles of both feet or palms of the hands, above the heel of the foot of base of the hand. The kidneys are central on both feet or hands, above the colon area. The reflected areas will be

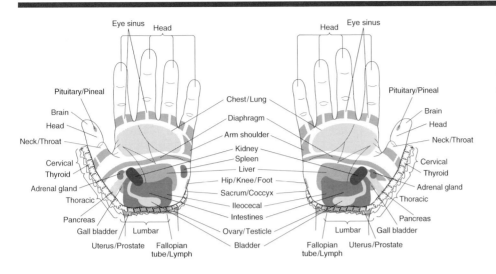

Figure 8-3

Many pressure points are located on the palm of the hand.

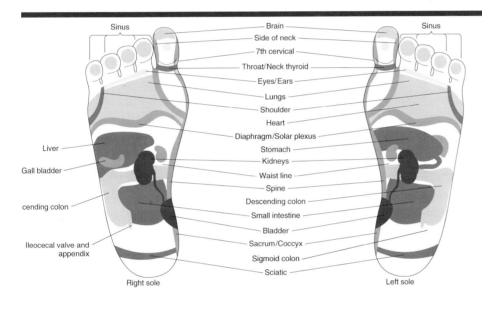

Figure 8-4

The feet contain more numerous pressure points.

specific to the corresponding kidney or area of the colon having a problem on the hand or foot of that side of the body (e.g., right kidney, right foot and right hand.) Discerning the reflex area for the organ is called "mapping."

Although this may seem farfetched to many, the results experienced by satisfied clients speak for the merits of reflexology. I can speak to that issue as a true doubter turned believer. Several years ago I decided to check out reflexology as a part of my instructor/writer research, so I looked for a qualified source of instruction on reflexology. After seeking referrals, I signed up for a certification course. The instructor was an experienced and licensed medical massotherapist who specialized in and taught reflexology. (I was the first manicurist in her class, actually. Usually, she taught graduate medical massage therapists.)

The first night was spend in defining reflexology and its history, describing the zones, and demonstrating on two students. I was one of those students and it proved to be very interesting. During that time, I was moving from one city to another—lifting and carrying. I was aggravating an old injury in my back and was chronically sensitive in that area. When the instructor placed pressure on the area of my foot that reflected that area, it was *very* tender and I recoiled slightly. She said, "Are you having some tenderness in your back?" Oh, was I! She worked on that reflex for an extended time, returning to it several times. When the treatment was over, I had *no* back pain and felt better and more relaxed than I had in weeks. Later in the treatment, she hit a second tender area and asked, "Do you have a thyroid condition?" Yes, she was right. And I knew I needed to have it rechecked because I'd been having symptoms lately. As the treatment proceeded, she mentioned the possibility of another chronic problem—and was correct.

After the class, I became a dedicated proponent for reflexology. I believe that although reflexology is a simple and harmless method of treatment, it can often produce amazing results for a client. If you are interested in the subject, even a doubter, one of the investigations you should undertake is experiencing the treatment from an expert reflexologist. It may be very enlightening.

Learning Reflexology

If you are interested in learning about reflexology, first read about it, as I suggested for aromatherapy. The many books on the subject are excellent and are written by experts in the field. Milady Publishing is a resource, as well as book stores and your library.

You should not assume, however, that buying or borrowing a book on the subject of reflexology and practicing from the pictures is enough to assume expertise in the technique. Books are a good resource for background on the subject, but they are not training; they are information.

Professional, hands-on training is essential for two reasons. First, there is a certain touch in reflexology; it is only learned through hands-on training, and clients who have experienced a reflexology treatment from an expert reflexologist *know* what that touch is. There is no substitute for a trained reflexologist to these clients and they will feel they have been defrauded. Second, an untrained reflexologist will not produce results for the clients, so they will see no reason to return. It is best for the salon and the professionals to pay the money for authentic training if they wish to offer the treatment and the clientele list to increase.

Accomplished instructors in reflexology will agree that hands-on training is necessary to learn the skill effectively. Courses typically have three sections:

- Lecture/demonstration
- In-class hands-on training.
- Applied reflexology to clients inside and outside of class.

Some courses have a final examination and a few require a clinical demonstration of expertise prior to receiving the certificate. A description of a credible course could be as follows:

> You will be taught theory, body mapping and point locations. Then, you will apply what you've learned to the clinical setting. There will be written examination scheduled after the last class. A certificate will be awarded to you upon successful completion of the course of study and 30 hours of applied reflexology outside the classroom.

(From Brochure, Reflexology Science Institute, Columbus, Ohio)

Seeking recommendations for a course is advised as well as asking the qualifications of the instructor and the amount of hand-on training contained in the course. Ask also if there is a requirement or suggestions in the class for purchasing specific brands of products. Product-driven courses are usually product-focused and may or may not provide sufficient training.

If you are interested in certification, contact one of the training organizations or search out a good course in your area. However, I suggest an interested professional attend a shorter survey course or a seminar for basic information and a demonstration of reflexology before signing up for a full certification course.

Reflexology and Governmental Regulation

No state at present requires a state certification before using the art of reflexology in massage. However, certain schools and specialists offer their own "certification." The value of these certifications is the knowledge provided the students during the required course and the dedication and professionalism it reflects to the interested client. The negative is the varying amount of quality of the teaching.

The regulatory agencies in some states consider reflexology an alternative medical practice. For instance, in Ohio at the time of this writing, continuing education classes in reflexology are not certified by the Ohio State Board of Cosmetology because it is considered medical.

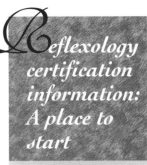

Reflexology certification information: A place to start

Foot Reflexology Awareness Association, PO Box 7622, Mission Hills, CA 91346. Offers information about training in California.

International Institute of Reflexology, PO Box 12642, St. Petersburg, FL 33733. Offers training and certification. (813) 343-4811

Laura Norman & Associates, 41 Park Avenue, #8A, New York, NY 10016. Offers training and certification. (212) 532-4404

Progressive Reflexology Institute, PO Box 22501, Kansas City, MO 64113. Offers training and certification. (816) 444-8779

Reflexology Research Project, PO Box 35820, Albuquerque, NM 87176-3820. (505) 344-5392

Reflexology Science Institute, 1170 Old Henderson Road, Ste. 204, Columbus, OH 43220. (614) 457-5783. Offers survey seminars, training and certification.

This seems contradictory and is certainly unclear because the practice of reflexology in salons is not prohibited, and the medical association does not support reflexology as an applied medical practice. Possibly all this will become more clear and consistent soon.

If you are considering practicing reflexology, I recommend you call your state regulatory board to ask their stand on its practice in a salon. Most states will classify it as a "harmless" massage technique and respond with "Go ahead. No problem," whereas others may have some official stand. You need to know what that is and adhere to the rulings. As alternative medicine becomes more regulated in the United States, we need to know what is officially accepted, rejected, or ignored as "harmless."

HAND REFLEXOLOGY

The feet have more than 7,000 nerve endings compared with fewer than 2,000 in the hands. For this reason, Eunice Ingham, a physiotherapist and founder of the National Institute of Reflexology, Rochester, NY, presently in St. Petersburg, FL, at the International Institute of Reflexology, felt it would be easier to access all the ten reflex zones through the feet and her detailed charts deal entirely with the feet. None of her charts, developed in the 1930s in a study of Dr. Fitzgerald's work, deal with the hands.

Many reflexologists disagree with her, however. Mildred Carter, noted reflexologist, author of *Hand Reflexology: The Key to Perfect Health*, and a student of Ingham's, says, "There is no portion of your wonderfully constructed feet which does not have its part to play in reflex massage. I will say the same for your even more important and intricately constructed hands. They also give you a unique way to health through the use of reflex massage."

Hand reflexology is similar to foot reflexology, except for the location. The theory is that by pressing and massaging specific points along the palms and fingers that relate to a corresponding organ or gland, the manicurist can relieve the congestion that is causing discomfort in these organs or glands. Hold your hand up in front to you, palms out, thumbs in the center, and look at them in the mirror. Think of them as "miniature bodies." Now you can map the pressure points according to those in Berit Nillson's chart.

Hand reflexology can be a positive adjunct to the practice of spa manicuring. A clientele is easily developed by giving away 5 minute samples. Two-minute samples are not adequate to get the results we need;

the client needs to see results to respond positively! Offer a client suffering from a headache a sample. It really works; she will feel the effects immediately and become a true believer. However, before you try this or any other reflexology, learn the skill properly, and practice, practice, practice. An accomplished reflexologist will sign up clients for the service with their first manicure after their sample! Or they will sit down at an appointment and say, "Can you add massage time to my appointment? I feel stressed."

How Reflexology Is Performed

Reflexology is performed with the thumb, the fingers, or a combination of the two pressing into the flesh over a specific reflex area for decongesting or stimulating. The thumb or fingers are pressed into the flesh at that spot deep enough to feel the bone or muscles underneath, then just slightly raised and "walked" to the next reflex point.

The motions are a "press and roll" or a "press and pull" motion. (Do not rub the skin.) This movement is described as "walking" the thumb or finger over the skin surface as the pressure points are sought. The reflexologist massages each area a specific time or number of repetitions and then moves on. (Fig. 8–5)

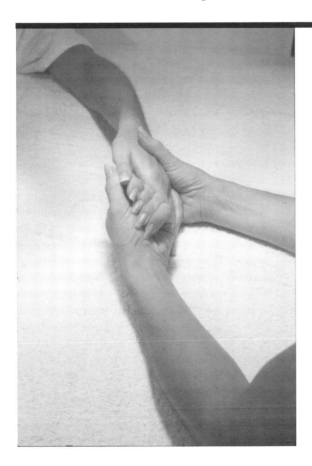

Figure 8-5

The reflexologist massages the hand to find the pressure points.

Reflexology should not be offered by a practitioner who has rough hands or tagged cuticles. The treatment is unpleasant from rough hands because the areas become sensitized during the treatment.

Some reflexologists believe that no oils or lotions should be used in performing reflexology, that they will interfere in the press and walk, through some essential oils may be appropriate. If the client's hands are moist, the reflexologist applies talcum powder to absorb the moisture. Others prefer to apply a light aromatherapy oil appropriately chosen. This is the decision of the professional.

Dedicated practitioners will say that accurate reflexology cannot be done with long fingernails; short nails will alleviate the possibility of scratching the client or offering a painful press when administering the massage. Others will say you can wear artificial fingernails and alter your hand positions to do the walking. My suggestion is that you take a survey seminar and try it so you can make an educated assessment of how your nails will affect your reflexology work. Your instructor will assist you in making the decision. My observation is that most professionals who enjoy extensive success in the art of reflexology do not have long nails.

A dedicated and informed spa manicurist will know that the quality of her massage techniques is significant to the success of her manicures and to the growth of her clientele. She will seek out expertise and refine her manipulations until she is confident they produce the desired results. (She will know they are because her clients will be saying: "Aaaaah!") Then she will proceed a step further into the perfection of specialty massages that she can enjoy giving and her clients will enjoy receiving during her spa manicures.

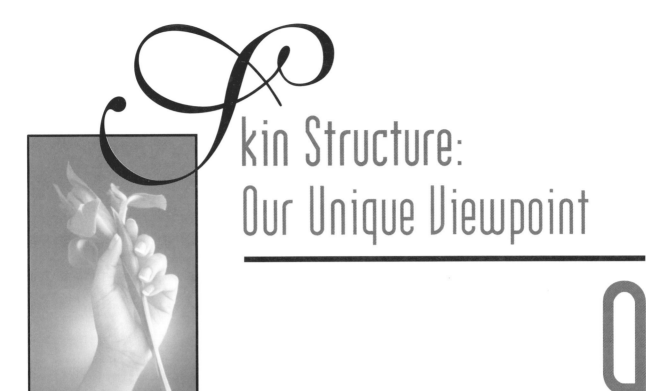

Skin Structure: Our Unique Viewpoint

9

OBJECTIVES

At the end of this chapter, you should be able to:

- Discuss the composition of the integumentary system.
- State the eight functions of the skin.
- Name the layers of the skin.
- Name the layers of the epidermis.
- Define collagen and elastin and describe their functions.
- Understand pores and follicles.
- State the appendages of the skin.
- Differentiate between sudoriferous and sebaceous glands.
- Differentiate between eczema and psoriasis.

When clients and beauty professionals think of skin care professionals, their thoughts go to *estheticians*. However, estheticians will soon share that reference with another professional group. With the implementation of the spa manicure and the upgrade of nail rooms, departments, and salons to nail spa, and manicurists to *spa manicurists*, the group called skin care professionals will include spa manicurists. These special manicurists are trained to include care of the client's skin during every visit and will become respected for this special knowledge.

To perform new skin care treatments within her new areas of expertise, the manicurist must be specially educated beyond their current training to support making appropriate decisions. This education will go beyond the structure of the skin as it is taught in nail classes currently. It will cover the unique structure and function of the skin on the hands and provide information that will provide support in the decisions she will make. These specially trained manicurists become a 'specialty within a specialty,' they are *spa manicurists*.

The manicurist who studies the structure and function of the skin will enjoy accurate, interesting, and correct care for her clients and will feel and portray professional confidence. She will be able to answer her client's questions and recommend treatments as a specialist in the area of skin care for the hands, arms, and elbows. This confidence and knowledge is experienced by the client, contributing to client loyalty and enjoyment of the service, and the manicurist experiences an expanded clientele, while fostering a new sense of respect in the beauty industry for her specialty.

INTEGUMENTARY SYSTEM

The skin is the largest organ of our body, a part of the integumentary system, which is composed of the skin, hair, nails, and the glands that serve them. It weighs 6 to 7 pounds, and the skin of an adult will cover 18 to 20 square feet, if spread out. Within 1 inch, according to *Milady's Standard Textbook for Professional Estheticians*, by Joel Gerson, it contains:

> 65 hairs
> 95–100 sebaceous glands
> 78 yards of nerves (70 meters)
> 19 yards of blood vessels (17 meters)
> 650 sweat glands
> 9,500,000 cells
> 1,300 nerve endings to record pain
> 19,500 sensory cells at the ends of nerve fibers

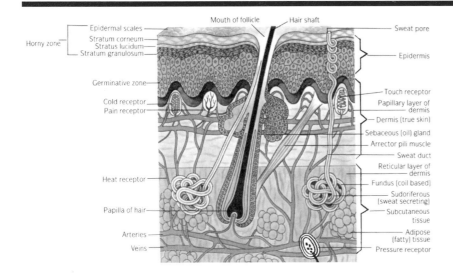

Figure 9-1

Diagram of the skin.

78 sensory apparatuses for heat

13 sensory apparatuses for cold

160–165 pressure apparatuses for perception of tactile stimuli

Healthy skin is composed of 72% water, 25% protein, and 3% fatty acids and minerals, optimally. Water is its most important element, as it is throughout the body, and its presence or lack in adequate amounts determines the skin's appearance and ability to maintain proper function.

The skin varies in thickness in different areas of the body. The thinnest area is on the eyelids. Thicker skin is present in areas such as the palms of the hands or soles of the feet. Situational thickening of the skin is caused by *intermittent pressure* in areas chronically exposed to pressure or friction for increasing protection. This thickening is known as a *callus* and is of special concern for manicurists and pedicurists because of the call for added attention and care toward their softening and exfoliation. *Continuous pressure* to these areas will cause *blistering,* a collection of clear fluid within or just beneath the epidermis, causing a raised elevation (a *vesicle*). Constant pressure prevents circulation to "feed" the tissue, causing the blister.

Manicurists must avoid treatment of blistered areas due to this collection of body fluids and the pain any contact will cause the client. Usually, blisters will force the injured person to remove the object causing the pressure, such as a working tool or a shoe, allowing the area to proceed through the healing process and return to a healthy condition. Generally, if a blister has not shown evidence of healing in 2–5 days, the client should be referred to a physician. If the object causing the intermittent pressure is not removed within a reasonable time, a deeper, ulcerative wound will develop, requiring treatment.

FUNCTIONS OF THE SKIN

The principal functions of the skin are:

1. *Protection* — The skin protects the body's delicate interior from injury and infection by preventing invasion through its outer layer, the epidermis. The epidermis prevents invasion of microorganisms, bars entry by most chemicals and gases, and lessens damage by ultraviolet rays. It can withstand tremendous physical pressure by objects before allowing a breakthrough.

2. *Heat regulation* — Normal temperature of the body (about 98.6°F, 37°C) is maintained by the activities of the blood and sweat glands in the skin. Heat is lost and the body cooled by the secretion of sweat on the skin surface, which evaporates, allowing cooling. Under cool conditions the blood vessels constrict, restricting the flow of blood to the skin while allowing maintenance of body heat as much as possible.

3. *Excretion* — Sweat glands excrete a liquid onto the skin's surface called *perspiration*. It contains salts and other waste products to be eliminated from the body.

4. *Sensation* — Millions of nerve endings in the skin respond to the sensory stimuli of heat, cold, touch, pressure, and pain, making it a sensory organ.

5. *Secretion* — The sebaceous glands in the skin secrete an oil called *sebum* for moisturization to the surface and layers of the epidermis. It also combines with perspiration secreted by the sweat glands to become the *acid mantle* present on the skin.

6. *Absorption* — The openings of the sebaceous (oil) and sudoriferous (sweat) glands allow the entry of certain drugs and chemicals into the body, such as fat-soluble vitamins A, D, and K and the drugs from the smoking cessation, birth control, and motion sickness patches. They also allow entrance of certain moisturizing and softening ingredients of specially formulated lotions, creams, and treatments.

7. *Storage* — The skin has limited storage functions, such as its storage of fat.

8. *Vitamin D synthesis* — Vitamin D is synthesized by the skin. Exposure to sunlight is necessary for synthesis to occur, however. Vitamin D acts on the intestinal and kidney absorption and reabsorption of calcium, a vital element to the survival and quality of life.

STRUCTURE AND HISTOLOGY OF THE SKIN

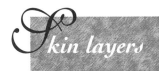

The skin is a thin, flat organ. Its physiology classifies it as a membrane —the *cutaneous membrane*. A membrane, in this context, according to *Webster's Encyclopedic Unabridged Dictionary*, is defined as "a thin, pliable sheet or layer of animal tissue serving as a limiting covering." It is made up of two layers, a thin outer surface layer, called the epidermal layer, or *epidermis*, and the inner, thicker layer, named the *dermis*.

Under the skin lies a layer of connective tissue called the *subcutaneous tissue*, or *hypodermis*. (It also may be referred to as *adipose tissue*.) This is not part of the skin, but connects the dermis with the muscle tissue below. Fat cells are found here, allowing it to act as a cushion between the muscles and skin. Its thickness varies with age, sex, and the general health of the individual, as well as with his or her weight. It provides energy from stored fat and helps keep the skin smooth, one of its most important functions in beautification of the skin. It provides the contour to the skin, also, defining our individual appearance as others see us.

The skin receives its nourishment and metabolic support from the subcutaneous tissue. The blood and lymphatics from this layer of tissue provide materials that support growth, nourishment, excretion, respiration and repair, all necessary activities of the cycle of life. Smaller branches of the blood vessels and lymphatics in the subcutaneous tissues are sent into the dermis to provide these materials.

Epidermis

The epidermis is the outermost layer of the skin. It is composed of two or three layers or strata in the thinskin areas, and of four layers or strata in thickskin areas. Some texts divide the fourth layer (stratum germativum) into two, allowing for five layers in designated areas.

All the layers work together in an ongoing cycle of life with the constant production of new cells and their push outward into each successive layer. Plump, live cells travel from the lowest layer of the epidermis to the outer layer, dying during their trip. They become increasingly flat and scaly and are sloughed off from the surface, to be replaced by other cells that have made the same journey and are also sloughed off. The process of sloughing dead epidermal cells is called *desquamation*.

This cycle of life, from the "birth" of an epidermal cell in a process termed *mitosis*, to the death and later sloughing of a cell, takes approximately 28 days in a young and healthy person. As a person matures, the process takes longer, possibly 32 to 40 days. This cycle of life is the

Skin layers

The arrangement of the skin as epidermis and dermis and the layers of each are important information the spa manicurist must know and understand to support professional decisions and recommendations.

basis for the recommendation by skin experts that skin care clients should have professional cleansings and other treatments on a monthly basis and should perform a daily home care regimen.

Production of the cells is ongoing and irregular, as is the travel through the layers toward the surface and the resulting desquamation. Therefore, in reality, no truly discernible layer is evident at any one time. However, the process is real and beauty professionals must know and understand how it works to effectively serve their clients. This understanding is more easily developed through a description of the process as though the cells were in discernible layers.

The "Layers" of the Epidermis. The epidermis is composed of four or five layers, according to how you label them. Named from the outside in, they are as follows:

1. *Stratum corneum* (horny layer)—The cells in this outermost strata of the epidermis consist of tightly packed, dead keratinocyte cells that are devoid of nuclei and cytoplasmic materials. They overlap at their margins resulting in a locking together of cells that have been converted into a water-repellent protein called *keratin*. Along with intercellular lipids that act as a natural adhesive to hold them together, they form an effective barrier until their time to be sloughed. They are continually being shed then replaced by new cells from the lower layers.

2. *Stratum lucidum*—This layer is composed of closely packed, transparent cells that light can pass through. Most of the skin of the body, the thin skin, does not contain stratum lucidum. It is present on the soles of the feet and the palms of the hands, areas of a spa manicurist's expertise. It is not present where there are hair follicles in the skin, leaving these two hairless areas to possess this layer. (Some texts will see this layer as the source for calluses in these areas.)

3. *Stratum granulosum* (granular layer)—Granules are visible in the cytoplasm of the cells of this layer. The cells are mature, flattened cells that are being killed by these granules of a protein called *keratohyalin*. They change into a hard substance and move on to the next layer, such as the stratum corneum. (This layer is missing in some areas of thin skin.)

4. *Stratum germinativum*—This layer in some charts is listed as two layers, represented as *stratum basale + stratum spinosum = stratum germinativum*. The *stratum spinosum*, the outermost of the two, is composed of live cells with spinelike extensions,

and is often called the prickle cell layer. These extensions join the cells. The *stratum basale*, composed of columnar-shaped cells, is called the basal layer by some persons. Only in this deepest innermost layer of the skin does mitosis occur. New cells are formed in this layer at approximately the same rate as the deal cells flake off the outer surface of healthy skin. Two types of cells are formed in the stratum basale: *keratinocytes*, keratin-forming cells, and *melanocytes*, the melanin-forming cells. This layer lies on the basement membrane, the membrane between the epidermis and dermis layers of the skin that cements them together in contact with the dermis below.

Melanocytes. Melanocytes are present in the stratum basale. They produce pigment granules, called *melanosomes*, which are passed on to keratinocytes in the stratum basale. Each melanocyte contacts several surrounding mitotic cells in the basal layer. (See Drawing) Their function is to absorb ultraviolet (UV) light and to absorb free radical molecules produced in the karatinocyte by that UV light. The melanosomes produce *melanin*, a coloring factor that is the basis of the color of our skin. This natural pigment serves as a protective screen against the harmful effects of the UV rays of the sun. Melanocytes are not more numerous in darkskinned people, they are more *active*, thus producing more pigment granules. These additional pigment granules produce more melanin and a darker skin.

A malfunction of the area where melanocytes are formed in the basal layer is responsible for the formation of age spots, darkened areas on the surface of the skin. The process of their formation is termed *hyperpigmentation*. (See Chapter 10.)

Dermis

The dermis, also called the *true skin*, is composed of a thick layer of dense fibrous connective tissue. The dermis contains an abundance of circulatory vessels (blood and lymphatic vessels) and nerve endings that are not present in the epidermis.

The dermis consists of two layers: the *papillary* and *reticular*. The papillary layer is named from the papillae arranged in curved, almost parallel ridges on its surface. Because the epidermis conforms to these ridges, the papillae are also reflected in the contour of the epidermis, especially on the tips of the fingers and toes. These ridges have a uniquely ridged pattern on each person and are the basis of fingerprints and toeprints. No two human beings have identical finger and toe prints, enabling us to be identified through these markings.

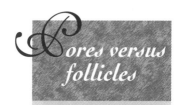
The reticular layer consists of a network of fibers. Most are collagenous fibers, or collagen, that provide the toughness to the skin. These fibers are the largest part of the dermis and provide structural support for the cells and blood vessels. They also aid in healing of wounds.

Collagen is responsible for the tone and suppleness of the skin. It is the condition of the collagen in the dermal layer of the skin that is reflected in the amount of lines and wrinkles in a person's skin. When the network of fibers weaken, the skin looses moisture and resiliency, and the appearance of lines and wrinkles becomes evident in the skin surface. This is a natural occurrence with aging but can be sped up and enhanced through damage, poor diet, and other factors.

Elastin, a protein present between the collagen fibers, provides the skin with elastic properties (rebound capability). Skin that has been stretched beyond its capability to recover will allow a tear in the dermis. The jagged scars are called stretch marks. An additional tear through the epidermis would make it a wound or a lesion open to the exterior.

Other structures with the network of the reticular layer are fat cells, blood vessels, lymph vessels, oil glands, sweat glands, hair follicles, nerve fibers, and *affector pili* muscles, involuntary muscles at the surface of a hair follicle that make our 'hair stand on end' when we are fearful or develop "goosebumps."

Appendages of the Skin

A definition of appendage is "that which is attached to an organ, and is a part of it." Appendages of the skin are the hair, nails, and sweat glands.

Hair. Hair performs no vital physiologic function in humans. Our body can be without it without any physiologic problems. However, only a few areas of healthy, normal skin are without hair, notably again the palms of the hands and soles of the feet. Sebaceous glands lubricate the hair by secreting sebum, an oily substance, into each hair follicle, the small tube from which the hair grows. A follicle is an epidermal projection from the dermis to the surface. (Fig. 9–1, p. 159) Hair is composed of tightly packed keratinized cells.

Nails. Fingernails are composed of heavily keratinized epidermal cells. They serve as protection for the fingertip and assist in grasping. Their visible part is called the nail body, while the rest of the nail, the root, lies in a groove hidden by a fold of skin, the cuticle, mostly posterior to the nail body. The nail bed is under the nail, a highly vascularized layer of epithelium, so appears pink through the translucent nail body. (Figs. 9–2 and 9–3)

Glands of the Skin. Three glands of microscopic size are *sebaceous*, *sudoriferous*, and *ceruminous*. Each has its own unique structure and function for perpetuating the cycle of life.

Sebaceous Glands

Sebaceous glands are little sacs that produce and secrete oil into hair follicles for transport to the surface of the skin (Fig. 9–4). There are at least two in each follicle. The semiliquid, oily substance, *sebum*, keeps the hair supple and the skin soft and pliant. It is composed of triglycerides and free fatty acids, wax esters, squalene, and cholesterol.

The mixture of sebum with perspiration from sweat glands, fatty acids, stratum corneum lipids, and amino acids present on the surface of the skin acts as a protective mantle, termed the *acid mantle*, against undue evaporation of moisture. A second function of the mantle is met by its slight acidity in pH; this property is one of our body's protections against undue microbial growth. Most microbes multiply poorly in an acidic environment.

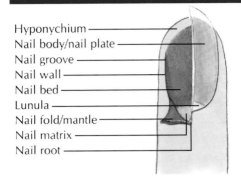

Hyponychium
Nail body/nail plate
Nail groove
Nail wall
Nail bed
Lunula
Nail fold/mantle
Nail matrix
Nail root

Figure 9-2

Diagram of the nail.

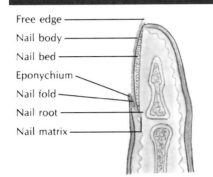

Free edge
Nail body
Nail bed
Eponychium
Nail fold
Nail root
Nail matrix

Figure 9-3

Cross section of the nail.

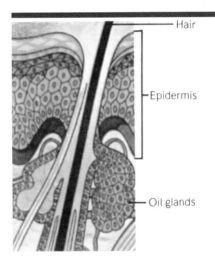

Hair

Epidermis

Oil glands

Figure 9-4

Sebaceous glands.

Preservation of the acid mantle should be a goal of the individual and her professional. Environmental attacks, highly alkaline soaps and cleansers, and overwashing the skin are the main reasons for damage to the mantle, enabling the undue evaporation of moisture from the skin. Dryness is the result. That does not mean that we should cut back on our handwashing and going outside. The acid mantle quickly recovers on healthy skin to the normal pH range of 4.5 to 6.0 following assault unless the damaging conditions or products are consistently repeated or the client is debilitated. (This ability to recover is called the *buffer capacity*.) It does mean, however, that the skin should be protected when in environmental distress, and the pH of products used on it should be balanced to enable cleansing while allowing minimal attack on this precious mantle. Repeatedly harsh stripping of the mantle can cause dermatitis, the invasion of disease causing microbes, and early aging.

Specifically, the lack of sufficient sebum on the surface of the skin is the cause of skin dryness. This lack can be due to removal of the secretion as mentioned or through suppression or reduction of oil production in the glands. Suppression or reduction can be due to systemic changes, such as aging or illness.

Sudoriferous Glands

Sudoriferous glands, or sweat glands, are the most numerous of skin glands. Two types are present, the *apocrine*, which are connected to and secrete their substance through the hair follicle, and the *eccrine*, which are not connected to a hair follicle. Eccrine sweat glands have a coiled base (*fundus*), a tubelike duct to carry the seat to the skin surface, and *pore*, (the opening to the skin surface). The apocrine glands are more active during emotional reactions, such as with fear, during tension, and during sexual arousal. The eccrine glands increase output during physical activity and higher environmental temperatures (Fig. 9–5).

The secretions from sweat glands play an important role in the *homeostasis* of body temperature (maintenance of balance). Evaporation of sweat has a cooling effect when body temperature is above normal. The secretions are watery and contain NaCl (sodium chloride, which produces the slightly 'salty' taste), potassium, urea, ammonium, and uric acid, as well as some other toxins and wastes such as heavy metals and organic compounds.

Ceruminous glands are a type of sweat gland located in the external ear canal. They secrete *cerumen*, a waxy, pigmented substance. They are of no interest to the manicurist function, but are noted as a type of skin gland.

Figure 9-5

Sudoriferous glands or sweat glands.

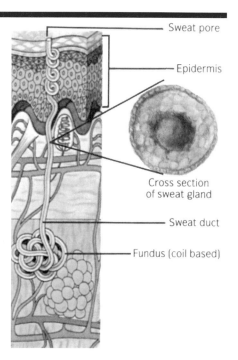

Sweat pore

Epidermis

Cross section of sweat gland

Sweat duct

Fundus (coil based)

Cutaneous Vascular System

Circulation of the blood through the skin layers serves two functions: (1) nutrition to and removal of waste from the skin, and (2) regulation of the body temperature by conducting heat from the internal structures of the body to the skin, where it is released by exchange with the external environment. These functions are carried out through two types of vessels: (1) the nutritive/excretory vessels (the arteries, capillaries and veins), and (2) specific vascular structures concerned with heat regulation, such as the subcutaneous venous network that can hold large quantities of blood. These structures react to changes in the metabolic activity of the body and the temperature of the surroundings, such as hot weather heating the skin causing vasodilatation and increased pumping of blood by the heart, allowing maximum heat loss. When the individual is exposed to extreme cold, vasoconstriction occurs, reducing blood flow and allowing minimal heat loss into the environment.

Relevant Inflammations

Inflammatory conditions, termed dermatitis, can be seen on the surface of the skin. These conditions may be caused by allergies, internal disorders, constant removal of natural lubrication, or environmental or occupational irritants. The skin may be of varying degrees of dryness and possibly sore, appearing reddened and raw. Manicurists see dermatitis often on their clients' hands and fingers and, less often, on their arms, elbows, legs, and knees.

Nonlesion inflammations can respond well to healing lotions that the spa manicurist applies and recommends, along with gentle scrubs and soothing treatments. **Note:** Clients with open lesions must be referred to a dermatologist for treatment. Skin care professionals are not to perform services on these clients.

A more serious condition often seen by a spa manicurist is *eczema*, an acute or chronic condition of dry or moist lesions. The skin may be itching and burning. It can be the skin's response to an allergy or internal disorder; the sufferer not under a physicians' care should be referred to a dermatologist. There is no known cure for the condition, but the client can be aided toward being more comfortable.

The term eczema is often used in referring to many different skin disorders that manifest in varying degrees of severity. Characteristic severe lesions are red, blistered, even oozing areas that itch painfully. The condition will come and go, be mild or severe, with no known reason for the changes.

Elbows and knees are often dry and in need of exfoliation. However, a more severe condition that the manicurist will see on those areas is *psoriasis*, a common, chronic, inflammatory disease; it can also be present on the chest, lower back, and scalp. The lesions are round, dry patches covered with coarse, silvery scales. These areas must be treated with gentleness because bleeding can occur if they are stretched or irritated. (The flexibility is gone from the skin's surface.) The disorder is not curable, but it can be treated by a dermatologist to make the client more comfortable.

Psoriasis may involve the nail matrix, plate, or nail bed, also in mild to severe forms. A client with mild involvement may never go for treatment because it can appear as just severely dry skin. Severe involvement can, however, cause intense pain and disfigurement of the nail area, so usually the client will go to a dermatologist for treatment in hopes of reversing the condition. As with psoriasis of the skin, the client with psoriatic nails must be treated with gentleness.

As spa professionals, we can perform manicures, treatments and programs, and recommend accompanying home care products that can aid our clients toward having beautiful and healthy looking hands. To do so, however, we must understand the structure of the skin and continually maintain a curiosity and knowledge of how new treatments will affect this structure. We need a basic knowledge about the skin, because it is especially relevant to us as spa manicurists, and a willingness to carry through with using that knowledge while nurturing a partnership of home care with our clients.

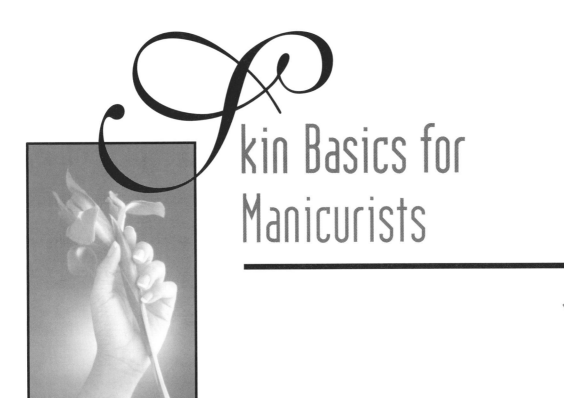

Skin Basics for Manicurists

10

OBJECTIVES

At the end of this chapter, you should be able to:

- Describe absorption of products into the skin.
- State the signs of aging of the skin.
- Define the differences between physical and chemical exfoliates.
- Describe how alpha hydroxy acid (AHA) works.
- State the benefits of AHA treatments.
- Compare AHA and retinoids.
- State the characteristics of dry skin and dehydrated skin.
- Describe the causes of age spots.
- Describe how moisturizers work.

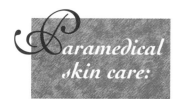

Paramedical skin care:

Most of us attended schools with curricula that concentrated on the mechanics of the manicuring service and the condition of the nail plate. When we start work in the salon, we know little about how we can improve the appearance of the skin, how the products we use work, and what, if anything, we can accomplish to improve the overall condition of the client's skin. For that reason, our manicures have perpetuated the status quo of the skin, at best, and we learned to dislike doing them a long time ago. Why bother, we thought. Following are basic precepts we should know to aid us in providing high-quality and correct services for our clients.

ABSORPTION OF PRODUCTS INTO THE SKIN

There are two levels of absorption of product, first, into the skin and then, into the cell. We will discuss the first level, absorption of products into the skin.

Previously, the skin was thought to be an impenetrable barrier, designed to protect our bodies from all invasion. Dermatologists openly discounted the possibilities of sufficient penetration of products for effective moisturization and repair by cosmetic formulations and, thus, any effectiveness of skin care.

With the development of *transdermal* medications, such as the smoker's patch, and the recently proven effectiveness of certain exfoliates and new moisturizers, new parameters have been defined for skin care. Cosmetic chemists used these new developments to enhance the effectiveness of their formulations, and a whole new world of effectiveness in cosmetic chemistry was born.

Because of current knowledge being inconsistent with information of the past, many clients are confused about how their skin absorbs professional and home care products. For that reason, spa manicurists must be able to clearly explain how products are absorbed into the skin.

There are two methods of penetration through the skin: directly absorbed or through the natural openings of the skin.

- *Natural openings* — Though the skin is an effective barrier for keeping out harmful substances, there are about 700 openings in every square inch of the skin which provide 700 points of penetration for effective products. These are our own sweat (sudoriferous) and oil (sebaceous) glands.

- *Direct penetration of the epidermal surface* — Certain substances can easily penetrate the surface of the skin via the intercellular materials. Example is vitamins, water-soluble substances with good lipid solubility, salicylic acids, and emollients. (Fig. 10–1)

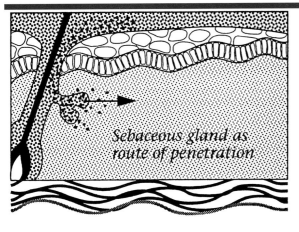

Sebaceous gland as route of penetration

Figure 10-1

Some substances like vitamins and water-soluble substances can penetrate the surface of the skin through intercellular materials.

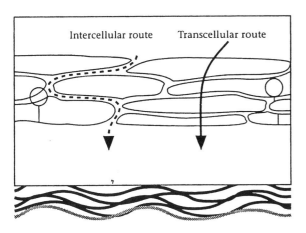

Follicle wall as route of penetration

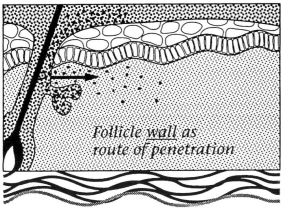

Intercellular route   Transcellular route

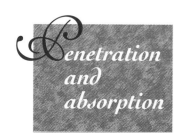

Penetration and absorption

Penetration and absorption are often described in separate and distinct terms by some skin care specialists. Penetration is described as when the product is taken only into the epidermis, while absorption is when it is absorbed deeper into the dermis. Penetration can aid the skin in moisturization and exfoliation, they say, while absorption can cause a change in the physical make up of the skin due to changes in the collagen and elastin, blood vessels, and nerves, as a result of the absorbed products.

Cosmetic chemists are producing new generations of effective treatments and cosmetics for our clients that focus on these methods of penetration. Appropriately formulated products easily transfer through the epidermis. Typical effective formulations consist of certain essential oils, emollients, moisturizers, vitamins, exfoliates, and other ingredients that are engineered to take advantage of these methods of transfer through the skin. When rubbed or applied to the surface of the skin, these ingredients are warmed by the temperature of the body, then lay on, exfoliate, penetrate, or pass through the skin, according to their functional design. After their penetration, they are absorbed into the cells in the layers and sublayers of the skin.

Contemporary masks, treatments, moisturizers, and other products are also formulated by cosmetic chemists with special ingredients that are especially selected for their ability to be absorbed into the skin and to nourish the cells.

Spa manicurists can contribute greatly to moisturizing, remineralization, and toning the client's skin and aid in healing and hydrating through professional treatments and recommendation of home care products and regimens. The professional educates her client on carrying through with the home care recommendations. The client does her part by purchasing and committing to the use of products in a specific home care regimen, guided by the spa professional's recommendations and directions. Together, the professional and client act as a team in meeting the client's needs.

AGING OF THE SKIN

We know that many persons go to great pains to hide the true age of their facial skin, but usually do not expend the same efforts on their hands. In our age-conscious society, many of us look at a person's hands for an approximation of their age. We can look to the hands for the truth. We'll say: "She has to be older than she says. Look at her hands!" (Fig. 10–2) The signs of aging on hands are as follows:

- *Fine lines and wrinkles* — Loss of elasticity in the dermis layer will allow the development of lines and wrinkles on the back of the hands, arms and elbow, right along with the facial skin. The skin will develop a crepiness, first, then later wrinkles. As we age, the subcutaneous layer shrinks and does not as effectively support the dermis and epidermis of the skin. (Fig. 10–3)

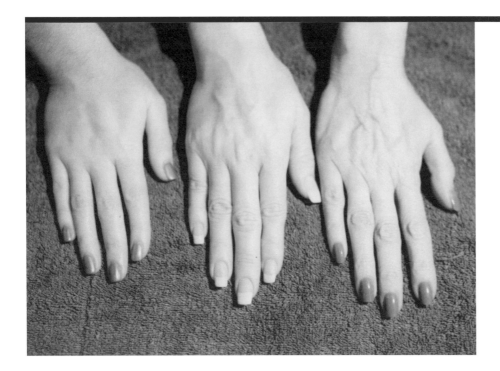

Figure 10-2

The hands can sometimes detect a person's age.

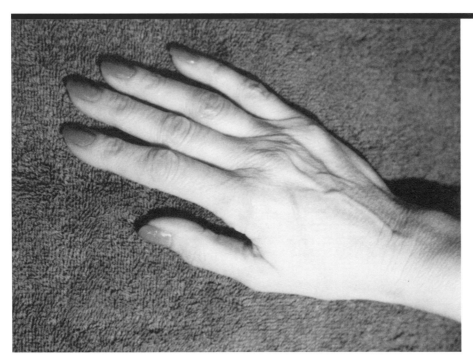

Figure 10-3

Fine lines and wrinkles develop from the loss of elasticity in the dermis layer.

- *Loss of tone* — The skin will appear "loose" or less attached to the bone structure of the hands. The skin will move easily when massaged.
- *Hyperpigmentation on the back of the hands and not on the palms* — These areas are most subject to the potent cause of the spots, the sun, more than most any other area of our body during

our normal activities, more so than our facial skin. The sun contains ultraviolet (UV) rays that damage the melanocytes thus causing them to darken, producing age spots as they move toward the surface of the hands. (Fig. 10–4)

- *Dry or dehydrated skin* — Sebum production from the sebaceous glands lessens with age, allowing the skin to become excessively dry. Hormonal changes also can cause chronic dryness. Dehydrated skin is caused by a lack of moisture in the lower layers of the skin.

- *Inflexibility of the bones and knuckles* — Mature knuckles may enlarge and hands may be less flexible. Conscientiously gentle care should be taken by professionals in preventing harm to the inflexible bones and knuckles of these clients. Older clients are very mindful of these changes in their hands. Because of them, they appreciate improvements in their skin through skin care treatments and the wonderful feeling of appropriate massages. (Fig. 10–5)

As spa professionals, we have an arsenal of techniques and products to aid the client in defying the ravages of aging in the area of our expertise. We must become educated in those efforts and in choosing and suggesting effective programs for appropriate clients. Of course, unless the client overtly requests help in making her hands look younger we must make our suggestions tactfully. We must also engage her as a partner toward meeting her goal.

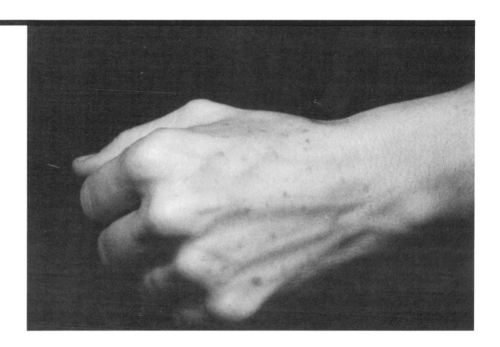

Figure 10-4

The sun's ultraviolet rays that damage the melanocyte cause age spots.

EXFOLIATION

Exfoliation is the most dramatic and therapeutic treatment a spa professional can offer a client whose hands show signs of dryness, aging, and the effects of the environment, illness, or neglect. For our purposes, it can be described as the releasing of dead cells from the surface of the skin. Appropriate products are available to us to enhance this normal activity of the skin and will make our client's hands softer and younger looking.

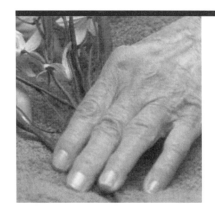

Figure 10-5

Professionals need to be extra-gentle to those clients with inflexible bones and knuckles.

Several different exfoliates are available to beauty professionals; others are restricted to use by dermatologist or plastic surgeons. Some will show wonderful results quickly and over time appear to be miracle products if used properly in partnership with the client in both professional and home care programs. Others are less dramatic but are appropriate for their particular clients.

The exfoliates that we use are physical and chemical exfoliates. Overall, the differences can be described through these criteria: how the exfoliate works, how deep it works in the layers of the skin, and whether it has residual effects (keeps on working after the treatment). Generally, physical exfoliates will work only on dead cells on the surface of the skin; chemical exfoliates may penetrate deeper and have residual effects.

Physical exfoliates remove the dead cells by mechanical means. Lotions with abrasives in them will be rubbed onto the surface of the scaly, dry skin. The abrasives will loosen and scrape the loose cells from the surface of the skin; only those that are loosely and superficially attached to the surface will be removed if the treatment is performed properly. Cells attached tightly with intercellular lipids will remain, allowing the skin to feel and appear healthier and smoother after the exfoliation. There are no known residual or negative side effects after use if the service is appropriately gentle.

Abrasive products such as almond, walnut, oatmeal, and silica scrubs are physical exfoliants. Oatmeal and silica are more gentle though effective than almond, walnut, and "natural abrasives" such as pumice, which may cause minute scratches in the stratum corneum. Sea salts are used on the hands, also, and are referred to as salt glow.

Enzymatic exfoliates are considered chemical exfoliates. Natural enzymes are applied and dissolve the dead cells off the surface of the skin. Those designed for our uses are designed to work on dead cells only. Many of them are from fruit enzymes, such as pineapple. Think of these enzymes as tiny "pacmen" that go along the surface of the skin "eating" the dead, scaly cells. The lower, attached cells will be ignored by these natural exfoliates, leaving a smoother skin with a healthier, softer appearance.

Enzymes speed the desquamation of the cells for a short time after the initial process and within a short distance into the layers of the skin so are thought to have a short residual effect toward continuing the desquamation of dead cells. Their function at the spa manicure table is to soften and prepare the skin for further and more efficient acceptance of treatment lotions and oils.

In the past, most enzyme peels were activated by water. Once the water is mixed into these produces they must be used immediately. They are distributed in powder form to professionals and are used under moist towels or with steam (professional vaporizer). If they are not kept moist, they crumble and are difficult to remove, and their exfoliation potential is compromised. For manicurists, the easiest application of these products is with a fan brush, then tightly wrapping the hands, arms, and elbows in a warm, not hot, towel. After the defined time, the towel is used to remove the product, and an exfoliated and smooth skin is revealed.

Enzymes are considered gentle through proactive exfoliants. However, there are potential allergies, so patch tests are advised prior to their use.

Enzyme products are being developed now as effective ingredients in exfoliant lotions and gel products. (These are much easier to use at the manicure spa table.) To be included in these vehicles for use, they have had to develop much more stable enzymes than have been thought to be previously possible.

Chemical exfoliates, such as alpha hydroxy acids (AHAs) dissolve the natural adhesive (intercellular lipids) that holds the dead cells onto the outer layers of the epidermis. This speeds the desquamation process, revealing healthier, smoother, younger looking skin in the process. They work in lower layers of the epidermis than other exfoliates. The speed of their effect is according to the strength of the chemicals. They have a residual effect in that they continue to work for an extended time in the affected layers of the skin, enhancing the desquamation process.

ALPHA HYDROXY ACIDS

The AHAs are nontoxic chemical substances that are derived from natural sources or can be synthetically manufactured. Natural AHAs have been used to beautify skin since ancient times. Stories are told of Cleopatra's obsession with milk baths, her form of AHA treatment, in her quest to soften her skin and maintain her youthful appearance. It must have worked because her beauty is legendary.

Modern cosmetic science has more specifically developed and refined the use of these acids for the benefit of women of our times. Now, they are considered "the skin care miracle of the 90s," though they have been used for centuries.

The AHAs are frequently part of cosmetic formulas. Termed "fruit acids," they do not all come from fruit, though most do. There are five that are frequently used in American cosmetics. Glycolic acid is from sugar cane; lactic acid is found in sour milk, bilberries, and tomatoes; malic acid is from apples; tartaric acid is from grapes and wine, and citric acid is from citrus fruits and pineapple. Many more AHAs exist and are effectively used in cosmetic formulations.

Each AHA has its own special properties. Lactic acid is known for being particularly good at moisturizing and gentle in exfoliating, whereas glycolic is the most effective at cell renewal, so these are the most frequently used in cosmetic formulations. Many times a combination of several AHAs is used in a product to take advantage of the benefits of each.

How They Work

As the skin ages, it slows in its ability to shed dead skin cells, causing the stratum corneum to appear dry, rough, and mottled, producing wrinkles and fine lines. AHAs work as exfoliates to remove dead cellular layers from the stratum corneum, leaving the skin fresher and brighter, and younger looking. They loosen the intercellular adhesive, termed *intercellular fluid, intercellular lipids,* or *interstitial fluid,* that holds the dead skin cells to the live epidermis, encouraging more rapid sloughing of these dead, keratinized cells off the surface of the skin. A more rapid turnover of cells results, bringing younger, more healthy skin to the surface. By applying professional strength AHAs to the skin surface for no longer than 10 minutes, the process of enhanced exfoliation of dead and sun-damaged cells will expose more youthful, healthier skin.

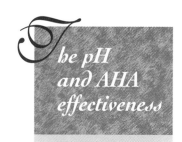

The percentage of AHA in a product is not the full story. The pH determines the exfoliation potential for an AHA. As ordinarily indicated by the pH scale, the lower the pH, the stronger the acid and the more exfoliation it will perform on the skin. Further, pH is exponential, meaning that a pH of 3 is 10 times stronger than a pH of 4. Most experts will say that the ideal pH for optimum results of an AHA is between 3 and 4.5.

Application of AHAs on the hands at 30% concentration or lower is considered an "intradermal procedure." This indicates it is a surface-repair treatment that causes desquamation of the stratum corneum only, and does not actively treat the lower layers of the skin (the dermis). Therefore, it is considered appropriate for use by manicurists. *As manicurists, it is important we do not use concentrations higher than 30% and insist on using products that are neutralized to a pH between 3 and 4.5.* These products will be effective, with consistent and programmed use, and will not cause obvious peeling, stinging or scarring for the client.

Many industry educators recommend lowering the highest percentage boundary to 20%. Others recommend a certification training program be required for use of chemical exfoliants while leaving the concentration at 30%. At present, however, the percentage is the decision of the spa owner/manager as is the amount of training, unless, of course, the laws or state regulations where the spa manicurist works require a lower percentage. This decision should be made according to the state laws, the extent of exfoliation training provided the spa professionals, their abilities/willingness to follow instructions, and the thoroughness and professionalism of their analysis steps.

Side Benefits of AHAs

The AHAs have wonderful side benefits. Studies show that, in addition to their exfoliation abilities, AHAs tend to stimulate the production of collagen and elastin in the dermal layer of the skin. Over time, a more toned, youthful appearance of the skin is noted. The skin is plumped up and appears thicker and more healthy. Fine lines and wrinkles are reduced as a result of the improved dermis, and pigmentation spots become lighter due to exfoliation. Pores (actually follicles) appear smaller. The surface of the skin is refined and retexturized. This only happens, however, with recommended, consecutive treatments and a dedicated home care regimen. "Occasionally" or "when I feel like it" does not work.

The use of AHAs is an opportunity for us to provide wonderful results for our clients. AHAs can provide great rewards in both increased income and client satisfaction. Clients can see dramatic results to conditions they formerly felt were to be just accepted as a part of life. However, using these products takes training and preparation to provide the services to their optimum result and to ensure the safety of the professionals and clients during their use.

Thinning the Skin

Questions estheticians and manicurists who use AHA and other exfoliates might receive from clients are whether exfoliates thin the skin and whether there is a danger in exfoliating too much. The professional should be able to respond to any questions concerning these possibilities with the facts.

In healthy, normal skin, gentle exfoliation enhances the natural release of already dead cells and thinning is not a probability. Actually, the skin has a positive response to exfoliation through a wonderful built-in mechanism in the basal layer of the skin; the skin responds to the natural desquamation process by stimulating mitosis (dividing to produce two cells from one) of the cells in the basal layer. Gentle exfoliation through sloughing or AHA treatments of the outer epidermal layers triggers the same response in the basal layer; exfoliated dead cells are replaced with new, healthy cells and the skin remains the same in depth. New, healthier, younger looking cells begin their journey toward the surface of the skin.

The stimulation of exfoliation of already dead cells toward the speed of normal younger skin is the goal in using exfoliates. *Overexfoliation* would have to be a conscious effort on the part of the professional, or, in the case of home care, on the part of the client. For a beauty professional to go past gentle is, of course, irritating, and the skin will quickly let the professional know when this has happened. When and if this happens, the professional *must* cease exfoliating immediately, and in response, the deeper epidermal layers will replace their missing layers in a healing process. A professional who insists on harsh exfoliations into the realm of irritation is unwise and can cause burns that may damage the deeper dermis, possibly causing what the questioner may be referring to as thinning the skin.

The basis of a beauty professional's exfoliation process is an exfoliation process causing enhancement of the natural process, only. Beauty professionals do not *peel*, proceeding into the lower dermal layers that can be permanently damaged, unless they are under the direct supervision of a dermatologist who is doing it for therapeutic purposes. That is when the skin thins.

Training Is a Necessity

Because most of our schools do not prepare us, as manicurists, for the use of AHAs, extensive and specific training needs to be obtained before you use them in a salon. Knowledge of the histology and physiology of the skin should be a specific requirement, and patch testing and safety must be emphasized. It is important the salon and professionals work closely with an AHA manufacturer or educator who is willing to provide specific training on the use of their product and the safety issues involved. Hands-on training is very important. If they are

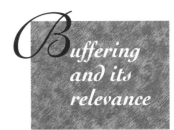

Buffering and its relevance

Many times labels will state that a product is buffered. For years, I felt somehow that this word meant it was a "less than" product, that it was "unnatural," that something negative had been added. To my surprise, on studying this process, I found it to be an important factor in maintaining its effectiveness. These are the facts about buffers:

Buffer—A substance that will aid another compound in resisting changes in pH in the presence of or when acids or bases are added. It acts to limit or prevent pH changes in that substance. Buffers are used in any product in which it is important to maintain a given pH level. Therefore, it is a "good guy," regardless of whether it is natural or not.

not willing to provide it, find a qualified educator or a manufacturer who will provide training.

As of this writing, the Food and Drug Administration (FDA) has not determined the highest percentage of AHAs for use in salons, but will pay close attention to incidents that carelessly cause damage or pain to clients in any decision they make. Incidences such as these could influence a decision toward rulings to remove the use of percentages that work effectively for our clients. A careful and caring professional will not take chances in the use of these products outside the parameters of safety. (Read the directions and listen closely during training!)

The exfoliators we use at our manicure table should bear instructions specifically written for use on the hands and feet of our clients. A patch test is performed, then they will be used weekly for a series of weeks. (Many professionals believe that the use of a high AHA lotion on the hands for a week or two prior to the initial treatment is an effective test for sensitivity.) After the initial treatment regimen, a maintenance schedule will be followed to stabilize the hands to "wonderful." A supportive home care program is essential to excellent results.

Patch Test

Performing a patch test is necessary but time consuming. The product is applied to a small area of the skin much the same as the actual treatment and left for the same amount of time as the treatment. (Read the directions.) For this reason, most spa manicurists will perform a sloughing treatment at the appointment when the client agrees to the series, and it is during this treatment that the patch test is done on the inside of the client's forearm. Then, the client is sold the home care products that are recommended and she uses them as directed until her next appointment when the AHA treatments will begin. The patch test and the use of the home care products will assure the professional that this client is not sensitive to the use of the product.

Some professionals believe that the use of the home care products for 1 to 2 weeks prior to the first treatment is enough to assure her that the client is not sensitive to AHA. They do not do an actual patch test. The policy on this issue is the decision of the management.

EMDA Information

The Esthetic Manufacturers and Distributors Association, a specialty branch of the American Beauty Association, has investigated exfoliates versus peels indepth to determine guidelines that can be safely used by skin care professionals. They determined exactly what guidelines we should follow to maintain safe usage and protection of our clients, while ensuring effective results. After their investigation, they agreed on a basic outline for usage among skin care professionals of these wonderful products and represented the professional beauty industry in legislative matters concerning this issue. For more information on this matter, EMDA can be contacted through the American Beauty Association, in Chicago.

AHA versus "Chemical Peels"

As we use them in our salons, AHAs are not "chemical peels" such as those used in the offices of dermatologists. The key term here is exfoliation. Exfoliation aids in the natural removal or sloughing of the superficial dead cells on the surface of the epidermis. In a *chemical peel*, a caustic substance is applied to the surface by a dermatologist to remove the skin's epidermis by liquefying (hydrolyzing) or removing many layers. It is an aggressive surface procedure and may involve removing portions of the more sensitive underlying tissue, the dermis, also. The procedure is painful, leaving the skin with a 'burned' appearance that must go through a lengthy healing process.

This procedure is done mainly to correct damaged skin surfaces and does not work well for aging tissue because it only slightly tightens the skin. (A solution of phenol or chloracetic acid, distilled water, and oil and liquid soap is often used in this procedure.) Conversely, exfoliation with an AHA according to directions will benefit aging skin. A smoother, younger looking skin will be the result, as well as producing a more toned skin and stimulating the production of healthy collagen and elastin in the dermis. It is not an invasive procedure—no pain or peeling when done according to directions.

AHAs versus Retin-A and Renova

Clients often want to know how AHAs compare with Retin-A and other similar retinoids. Retinoid is a term used to generally refer to products derived from vitamin A, which is added in strengths that usually require prescriptions from a medical doctor. In truth, both AHAs and retinoids slow down skin aging and help acne problems on the face, but they perform very different actions on the skin. Retinoids work by dissolving the epidermal layers and creating a rapid growth process. In this process, extreme dryness, cracking, and irritation can result. It improves the blood flow, which can encourage collagen growth, but it also may produce a harsh red skin on the user. Also, the client must stay out of the sun because even short exposure can produce a severe sunburn. Seldom are retinoid products used on the hands due to the difficulty in controlling their exposure to the sun.

Fruit acids are more gentle products. These AHAs enhance desquamation, without aggressively peeling the outer layers of the epidermis. Used properly, no extreme dryness or irritation occurs. The skin has a natural glow that is revealed when the dulling layer of old skin is encouraged to desquamate from the surface, not the reddened appearance that is defined by retinoid treatments.

The AHAs are perfect for the hands. They do not make the skin sun sensitive so they can be used daily and the client can still go out in the sun without undue concern about sunburn. A sun block must be used, of course, to prevent further sun damage and overexposure to the rays of the sun, and it is our duty to encourage our clients to use it routinely. The constant exposure of their hands to the environment requires sun block.

BETA HYDROXY ACID

Beta hydroxy acids (BHAs) have been used by dermatologists for decades to treat acne, dandruff, psoriasis, and other conditions. The activating chemical is *salicylic acid*, a chemical of multiple uses in our lifestyles. Aside from its usage in prescriptive treatments, forms of it are in more mundane over-the-counter (OTC) products such as aspirin (acetylsalicylic acid); commercial pastes, patches, and brush-ons for corn removal; retail acne medications; wart removal medications; dandruff shampoos; and more. Its effects are analgesic (pain relieving) and anti-inflammation in aspirin; in the OTC skin and scalp medications the targeted activating property is cell exfoliating.

The cell exfoliating properties of salicylic acid have come to the attention of skin care formulators for reducing wrinkles. Recently, very low concentrations of BHA are being used as additives for a few retail beauty products for gentle and effective exfoliating of the cells in the stratum corneum. Some professional-line skin care developers are considering BHA the next magic ingredient for anti-aging and cell renewal. In certain concentrations they are proving to be more gentle while producing better results than AHAs. Several skin care companies are marketing BHA products.

Professional companies are taking development of BHA products more slowly than the retail companies though many formulations are available now. BHA can be very irritating in certain concentrations and the potential for allergies is much higher than with AHAs. Also, at a pH of 4 or 5, the product becomes inactive; a pH that is too low is irritating. The ideal pH for BHA exfoliates is about 3.0.

The most important advantage of BHA as an exfoliant is that it has shown an additional capability for cleaning out clogged pores through activating/enhancing the exfoliating of surface cells inside the follicles, not only on the surface of the epidermis as with AHAs, and the surface exfoliation properties are excellent at lower concentrations. The potential, with this capability, is the shrinkage of the pores themselves, a desirable effect in anti-aging and surface renewal that has not been met by AHAs.

Professional companies are testing/perfecting the use of both AHAs and BHAs in combination for producing possibly the best results yet in skin renewal. AHAs will be used for their wonderful moisturizing and renewal of the lower layers of the skin, while the capabilities of the BHA to cleanse and shrink the pores and gentle slough the surface will be added.

A further consideration is that lower percentages and lesser amounts of the inexpensive BHA can be used in the cosmetic formulation, allowing the product to be less expensive to produce. When cosmetic chemists feel these potentials can be safely and effectively reached, we will see more professional products available with salicylic acid in them.

Public information of the possibilities of salicylic acid as a miracle wrinkle remover has a serious negative potential, however. Application of this chemical to the surface of the skin by the uninformed masses in home remedies can produce devastating burns that are as severe as if a flame were used on the skin. Can you imagine uninformed persons plastering pastes of aspirin and water on their skin for inexpensive wrinkle reduction? The thought is scary, but a possibility to be considered by manufacturers eager to shout "Salicylic Acid Will Make You Look Young!"

Not as potentially dangerous, but *very* drying would be the application of globs of teenage OTC acne medications that are salicylic acid based onto the skin of the frugal but wrinkle-hating masses. Professional formulas will be more gentle and more moisturizing.

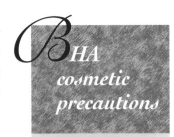

BHA cosmetic precautions

Precautions to be noted in recommending BHA cosmetics for a client are its potentials for irritations and allergies. Although BHA products will not cause any problems for the majority of clients; those with cosmetically sensitive skin should be use tested, meaning the product should be used on a small area exactly in the recommended regimen for a few days or even a few weeks before widening its scope to the full area of use.

Clients who are prone to allergies must have a cosmetic patch test for sensitivity. If no reaction is noted, the client can assume she is not sensitive to BHA.

Clients who have allergies to aspirin or other salicylates should not use cosmetics containing BHAs. Cosmetic products with salicylic ingredients will typically be sunscreens, acne treatments, and exfoliates.

MOISTURIZATION

Dry skin is not as simplistic as it appears in that it can actually be *dehydrated* skin or a combination of dry and dehydrated skin. A skin care professional must understand the appearance of the two and their causes to discern what treatment and home care should be recommended to their clients. This understanding is especially important to the manicurist because many of her clients will less actively address problems with their hand than their faces unless their spa professional educates them fully to the need and correctly defines the methods for effective treatments and home care.

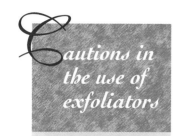

Cautions in the use of exfoliators

The horny layer (stratum corneum) is there to protect the deeper layers of the skin. Any exfoliation treatment removes a part of this protective layer. It is replaced quickly, yes; but it is removed. Exfoliates also temporarily remove the acid mantle. For these reasons, the skin should not be in direct sun or cold or wind and waxing or other depilatories should not be performed for at least 24 hours.

Exfoliation should not be done on the skin of clients who are using retinoids or Accutane or are sunburned. Also, clients with sensitive skin should not be exfoliated, so a patch test should always be done to determine a new client's sensitivity level to the product. In considering a bomelain-based enzyme product, check for an allergy to pineapple.

If intense stinging or burning occurs during the application or treatment, the product should be neutralized immediately. Essential oils should not be used before or after the exfoliation.

Using exfoliates is a responsibility that should only be accepted after full education and supervised practice of the procedure. Cautions should be considered with every client.

Dry skin can be a surface condition of lacking oils (intercellular lipids) and usually is caused by environmental factors. As manicurists, we have all seen it on bartenders, moms, nurses, and many other clients whose hands are constantly stripped of the natural protection of oils present on the outer layers of our skin. They can be exposing their hands to repeated washings, solvents, cold weather, wind, and various other factors that strip these oils. A working description of dry skin is scaling, flaking, roughness, sometimes cracking, and redness. The texture of the skin is characterized by fine wrinkles on the surface and degrees of roughness. Generally, dry skin can be dealt with by salon treatments, an emollient home care regimen, and some redesign of the client's lifestyle.

Dehydrated (aging) skin is more complex than dry skin. The telling characteristics of dehydrated skin are pronounced lines and much less elasticity. However, the symptoms can be similar to that of dry skin along with those of dehydration. The wrinkles and creases indicate damage to the dermis of the skin that will not be resolved by the typical moisturizer. Their presence indicates a change in the collagen/elastin matrix in the dermal layers of the skin.

The causes of dehydrated skin are generally from within. Typical causes may be chronic dieting, chronic exposure to the sun, insufficient intake of water, and illness. For some reason, the dermal layers of the skin are not supplying sufficient moisture to the epidermal layers, and the underlying tissue is not providing the needed support. It begins to look older, with many wrinkles, and does not have the smooth, plump appearance it should have. It may be less elastic and will not seem as strong and resilient.

Properly formulated moisturizers can address these conditions. They provide the topical lubrication that the outer layers of the epidermis need to address the surface dryness and ingredients that enhance the moisture retention of the layers. They cannot, however, fully "cure" the problem because it is usually perpetuated until the deeper cause is resolved.

The moisturizing ingredients used in cosmetic formulations to address these conditions can be classed into two types of materials: lipid moisture barriers and humectants.

Lipids or Fats and Oils. The skin cells of the epidermis and dermis are held together by *intercellular lipids*, oils that act as a barrier, retarding water loss from the skin. The fact is that the main job of a moisturizer is to hold in the moisture that is already there.

Intercellular lipids need water to do their work. When they are deprived of this moisture on external (dry skin) or internal (dehydrated) levels, they become incapable of doing their job. The skin begins to appear dry and wrinkled, the cuticles become hardened and flaky, and hangnails develop. Overall, the skin is less elastic and ages quickly.

Hundreds of fats and oils act as simple barrier-type moisturizing ingredients. The most mentioned are mineral oil, silicones, isopropyl myristate and petrolatum. Natural oils are being used more often because of their excellent barrier moisturizing qualities as well as their absorption capabilities. They far surpass the absorption of these old ingredients that were excellent barriers, but whose molecules were far too large for much absorption and use in the lower layers of the skin. There are hundreds of natural oils, also. Among them are evening primrose oil, orange roughy oil, aloe oil, borage oil, sesame oil, sweet almond oil, squalene, and avocado oil. Vitamin E is also an oil that has excellent moisturizing qualities.

Lipids have the added potential of enhancing healing the outer barrier layer of the skin. Without the healing property, the other benefits of lipids would be unsuccessful in moisturizing the skin.

Humectants. Moisturizers are complex formulations that aid the body in using its own hydrating mechanisms to maintain the needed balance of fluids at the cellular levels of the skin. Aiding the cells to attract and hold water is the job of the second type of moisturizing ingredient, *humectants*, additives that have the ability to draw moisture from internal and external sources and hold it to themselves.

One such attracting chemical is *hyaluronic acid*, which occurs naturally in our body but can also be produced synthetically for use as an ingredient in moisturizers. When formulated into a moisturizer, one molecule of hyaluronic acid can attract and bind to itself up to one million molecules of moisture. Therefore, applying a moisturizer with a good humectant ingredient to a dry skin area can draw needed moisture there while holding it on the surface or inside the skin.

HYPERPIGMENTATION

We are all born with clear, smooth, even textured skin with the "baby's bottom" appearance we refer to in describing perfect skin. However, after decades of exposure to environmental damage, this surface shows damage to the lower layers of the epidermis with brown spots and discolorations. This slow process does not just show up one day, though

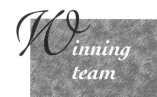

awareness of the presence of the spots may be sudden. One day a client may see them and may even become obsessed with their presence. Actually, it takes a long time for these spots to develop, it can be from damage to the skin as long as 20 years ago.

Those darkened areas can be anywhere on a person's skin—hands, face, legs—anywhere that is exposed to the ravages of the rays of the sun. However, the places that annoy clients the most are the hands. Those dreaded age indicators are right out there for anyone to see at all times. This is not to say that the ones on the face do not bother clients, but those can be covered with makeup. Spots on the hands will not be, usually, and are out there telling the truth about their age, or worse, are making them look older than they really are.

Hyperpigmentations are usually on the back of the hands and not on the palms. These areas are most subject to the potent cause of the spots, the sun, more than most any other area of the body during normal activities. The sun contains UV rays that damage the melanin-producing cells, melanocytes, deep in the layers of the skin, thus producing the darkened areas.

Dermatologists use many methods for removing hyperpigmentations immediately; some are rather new, such as the use of lasers. Lightening products can also be used, though they are slower and are termed lighteners because they never completely eradicate the severely darkened spot. Many clients choose them over the more invasive procedures, however.

Hydroquinone, the most usual ingredient used in lightening products, is the only product presently approved by the FDA for skin bleaching. Other products such as Kojec and/or licorice rood are normally used. In reality, these products do not actually lighten or bleach the skin. Instead, they reduce the production of *melanin*, the pigment that produces the color deep in the layers of our skin. UV causes damage to the *melanocytes*, the producers of the color, resulting in *hyperpigmentation*, a surplus of color. By reducing the production of melanin, the resulting color of the cell is lighter, or at least not hyperpigmented when it comes to the surface.

Home care for a client concerned with hyperpigmentation *must* include a sunscreen or the treatments will be futile. A sunscreen is necessary after the peel to protect the exposed layers of the skin from further sun damage and the resulting further hyperpigmentation of the lower cells. SPF 15 is to be applied every day before exposure to the sun. Further applications of the SPF product should be done after each handwashing. For that reason, manicurists need to seek out and recommend a purse-sized product applicator.

I recommend a small area applicator, as the one pictured. (Fig. 10–6) The use of a lotion lightens the entire area, including the background skin of the age spots. The spots will lighten, but the lightening to the same degree of the background skin will defy illustration of the lightening of the age spots. The same contrast between the skin and the background skin will be maintained. Because it is done over a span of time, the client will not "see" the lightening of the spot. Application with a small area applicator will allow the lightening to be seen as only the spot will be lightened.

To this time, SPFs have not had much role in a manicurist's professional care. This should change in our routine home care recommendations. If we truly care about the future appearance of our clients' hands, we should be recommending they use SPF 15 or above *every day, all day,* on their hands. They are getting sun damage on their hands even through the car window while they drive.

As of this writing, professional product manufacturers are developing some great new moisturizing hand lotions *with SPFs* for our clients. These are wonderful additions for meeting the needs of our clients.

In summary, the three ways moisturizers aid the body in using its own hydrating mechanisms to maintain the needed balance of fluids at the cellular levels of the skin layers are acting as a barrier against the escape of water from the surface of the skin, by repairing the skin's natural barrier to the environment so the body's internal healing processes can do their job, and by attracting water to the dry area.

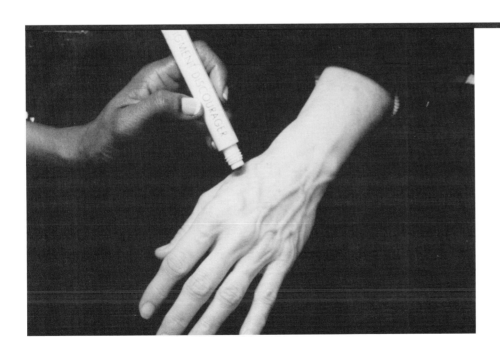

Figure 10-6

Age spots can be lightened with the use of product in a small applicator.

Exfoliation is one of the basic skills that skin care specialists must know when treating clients in the new millennium. This has become true also of manicurists as the clients widen their improvement expectations to the hands. Aging and its ravages, such as hyperpigmentation, are "Baby Boomer" enemies, and we are one of their defenses. We must understand the processes to be able to give them their immediate improvements over these ravages that they expect.

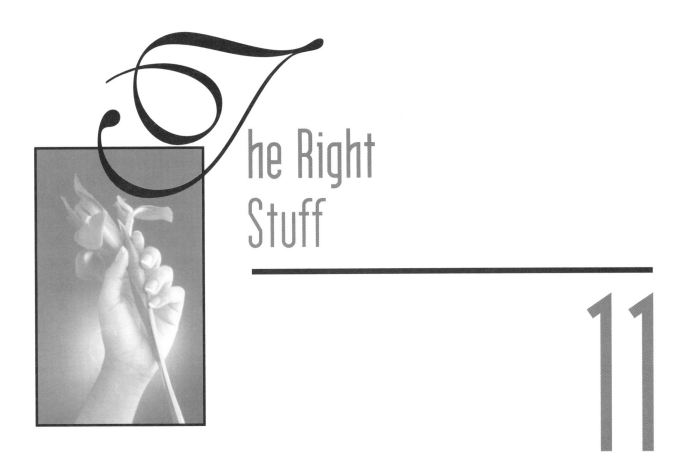

The Right Stuff

11

OBJECTIVES

At the end of this chapter, you should be able to:

- Purchase the basic utensils for spa manicuring.

- Discuss carrier and essential oils.

- Name the five types of lotions.

- List the four uses of mineral oil in lotions.

- Purchase a balanced menu of lotions for the professional and retail menu.

- Discuss the types of cuticle treatments.

- Choose professional and home care cuticle treatments.

- Purchase quality post-service products, such as top and base coats.

- Develop accessory products to meet the needs of the clientele.

A professional must have proper equipment and supplies to perform her skills well. The basics I consider essential for spa manicure professionals are listed below. Experience in performing the services will dictate others a spa professional might wish to add. Tools are ultimately the choice of the professional and nail spa, as dictated by the services they wish to provide. The list will not include large equipment, such as the table and paraffin bath. (Fig. 11–1)

UTENSILS AND SUPPLIES

Antiseptic hand scrub
Manicure scrub brush (nylon)
Polish remover/removal materials
Table/hand towels
Cuticle lotions/cremes
Treatment and home care lotions
4"x 4" treatment squares
"Plastic pusher"
Metal pusher
Ruby stone and shaping stone
Manicure nippers

Cuticle oil
Paraffin
Plastic bags or wrap
Nail files/emeries (sanitizable
    or disposable)
Base coat
Polish
Quick-drying top coat
Drying equipment
Home care products

Figure 11-1

The spa and professional generally choose the tools they want according to the services they provide.

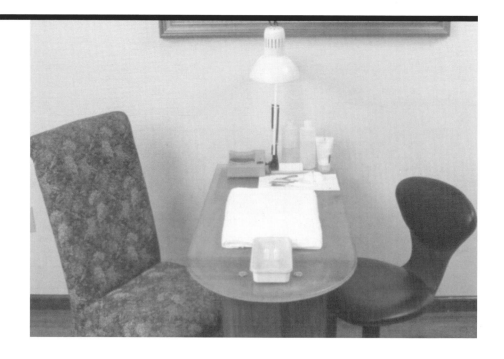

Spa Manicuring for the Salon and Spa

The choice of quality products and utensils will be significant to the success and efficiency of the services.

EQUIPMENT AND SANITATION

A beauty professional must consider sanitation procedures when assembling equipment, utensils, and supplies for spa manicuring. Metal implements must be stainless steel or high carbon steel to prevent corrosion during the disinfection process, and the manicure brush must be nylon to permit disinfection (natural hair brushes cannot be disinfected). For efficiency, a busy nail spa professional will need at least three sets of reusable implements (marked with an asterisk in the supplies list) for manicuring. Fewer sets will foster short-cutting in proper disinfection routines and cut efficiency. These implements will be used as following:

> One set will be in use
> One set will be in the sanitation system
> One set will be ready for use.

Such a routine will make it possible to have clean, sanitary implements always available for each client and the professional will have fewer concerns.

PROFESSIONAL PRODUCTS

Generally speaking, the only difference between professional and home care products in spa manicuring is the size of the containers, with the exception of professional exfoliation products and treatment masks that are not sold as home care products.

The ideal criteria for well-chosen professional products are:

1. The ingredients will be of high quality and of benefit to the client.
2. Collectively, the products will cover every possible client need that the professional chooses to address in her services.
3. The products will not usually overlap in their purpose, wasting money or testing time on products that duplicate clients needs. The exception may be the aromatherapy lotion, which is also moisturizing and will usually overlap the inventory and service needs of the professional and retail emollient and moisturizing lotion.

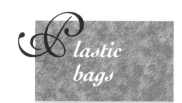

Plastic bags

The thin and malleable plastic used for encasing the hands and feet during treatment services is very important to the effects of the treatments. I suggest that the big bags used to cover the perms in the hair department are not beneficial for use in the manicure department. They are too large, which prevents them from holding the heat to the hands and feet of the client, and are too short, which prevents the arms (and legs) from getting the best benefits of treatments. Worse, it is obvious to the clients that they just are not appropriate—they just do not feel right. The person in charge of product acquisition should find thin but long, appropriate width plastic bags from a commercial bag company. They should come in bulk, be inexpensive, and do the job that should be done. The thickness should be similar to the hair bag, however; thin is better because they are malleable but still hold in the heat. The effort is worth it, if just for the enhancement of the treatment and for the appearance of being appropriate for the service.

4. They will mesh together as a "product team" that can be used purposefully in the services.

5. The product manufacturers will provide support with information and education on request. If required, the material safety data sheet is provided, although few manicure products require one.

6. The products will be easily used and fully understood by the professional.

7. The products will be accompanied by home care sizes for use by the clients in perpetuating their therapeutic effects.

8. The professional products will be priced within the niche of the salon and the home care products will be priced within the niche of its clientele.

9. The product company has sample sizes of the home care products.

Choosing products is time consuming and tedious. Methodical testing should be performed after the products are obtained and before their permanent incorporation into the salon regimen and client care. The testing criteria are chosen according to the wishes of the professionals, the desired results for the clients, and the profitability parameters of management. The performance criteria should be *written down* for each product and the performance measured and recorded; then when all the products are tested, a decision is made according to these written judgments. The criteria will be properties such as results, "feel," (how they feel on the skin and in use), aroma, and ease of dispensing, among other things. The tests should be performed on *testing clients*, not paying clients.

Cuticle Pushers

Wooden cuticle pushers must be removed from use in the salon unless they are thrown away or given to the client after use. They are *not* sanitizable. The spa professional can use a stainless steel pusher gently and wisely and purchase sanitizable plastic cuticle pushers for use when appropriate. (Some are not sanitizable.)

LOTIONS: OUR PRIMARY PRODUCT

With traditional manicuring, we usually had one lotion for use on our clients; a heavy, sticky lotion that rarely produced results for the client for more than an hour, though it was great for the massage. It was designed to use in the manicure heater for the hot oil manicure and for use during the massage. Now there are hundreds from which to choose and they no longer contain the same old ingredients.

These newly formulated lotions are the very basis of spa manicuring. The choice of the right lotions for a client's service and home care will enhance the table service, maintain the manicure effects between appointments, and improve her skin.

Designing a lotion can be a work of art with the needs of a special client in mind or a tube of junk that has no purpose but happens to feel good for a short time. We must recognize the difference, with our clients' benefit as our focus. Actually, there is no perfect lotion. Each has its own special ingredients and its own effects and purpose for use on the skin if it is a good design.

As we attempt to make the best choice of lotions to meet the needs of our clients, we must depend on the ingredients and the claims on the label as our sources of information. If we need help in translating that information, it is available, written in language we can understand; several books have been written to help us in interpreting what we need. I suggest that the spa resource manager or nail spa manager purchase a cosmetic ingredient book and an aromatherapy book to help discern a lotion's capabilities before purchasing it. When I am looking for a lotion, I carry my books and look up any ingredients listed on the labels about which I have no knowledge. (I am not a cosmetic chemist and do not aspire to be!) These books give me valuable information as to the uses of the lotions and, if they do not give me the answers, they point me to questions I need to ask the manufacturer. These books have saved me considerable money, frustration, and valuable space on my professional and home care shelves. Best of all, I have improved results with my client care.

By law, the Fair Packaging and Labeling Act of 1966, a list of ingredients must be available to the *retail* purchaser, either on the container, box, or piece of paper that accompanies the product. (Fig. 11–2) The ingredients are listed according to their percentage by weight in the product and must be readily available for the consumer to read. The designed purpose of the product should be stated on the label, as well as in their marketing claims, (though this is not required.) It is interesting that professional-only products are not required to carry this information, though most do, as a service to their nail professional consumers.

Ingredients

Providing a few paragraphs in this book about cosmetic ingredients for lotions is almost dangerous, but an introduction is important to the information that will follow. These paragraphs will introduce carriers and essential oils, hoping the spa resource person will seek further

Figure 11-2

Ingredients are listed
on back of product.

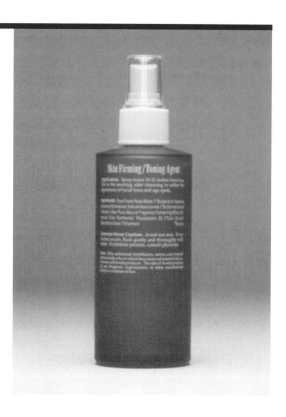

information to make him
or her more knowledgeable
in the choices of products.

Carriers. Carriers are
exactly what their names
indicate—they provide a
vehicle or base for other
ingredients, such as the
essential oils, to be carried
to or into the skin. They
will usually be one of the
first two ingredients listed, although water is the
first listing in many formulations. Examples of
carriers are mineral, aloe,
almond, sunflower, saf-
flower, and grapeseed,
among a great number. If
a purchaser knows them
well, these oils can indicate to her the best use of the oil or lotion in
performing a service. (If she does not, she should buy that book and
look them up!)

Carriers are oils and most have a therapeutic value aside from their
work-horse attributes, and most designers of quality lotions will
choose one that has this capability. Some examples follow.

- *Mineral oil* is a clear, odorless oil derived from petroleum.
  It is non allergic and is used in cosmetics in a refined state.
  It can be comedonic in some grades, which is of course no
  problem for a manicurist. Its best quality may be its ability
  to form a barrier for the skin's natural moisture and its
  wonderful slippage in a massage. It can be absorbed into
  the skin when it is the highest refined grade available.

- *Aloe vera* is an emollient and film-forming gum resin with
  hydrating, softening, healing, antimicrobial, and anti-
  inflammatory properties. It is highly moisturizing, regulates
  the moisture in dry skin, and is one of the most widely used
  due to its excellent properties and low cost. It has excellent
  penetration, supplying moisture directly to the tissues, but
  this penetration is highly dependent on the correct concentration of the ingredient, which is a problem that is usually

undetectable on the label. (This may be a question to ask the manufacturer.) Concentrations over 50% have shown to increase the blood supply to the area of application.

- *Grapeseed oil*, an excellent carrier, is moisturizing and has nourishing properties.
- *Safflower oil* is considered hydrating to the skin. It is soothing and healing to the skin, containing lecithin, linoleic acid, fatty acids, and caroteniods.
- *Almond oil* is an excellent emollient, making the skin feel elegant and promoting great spreadability to the product.
- Avocado oil is an excellent emollient and soother, is bacteriocidal, and may mobilize and increase the collagen of connective tissue.
- *Macadamia oil* is an emollient carrier with excellent spreadability and penetration properties. It has a nice, smooth, nongreasy aftereffect, and is gentle to the skin. Its structure is similar to the skin's sebum. It especially benefits maturing skin due to the palmitoleic oil content and is a wonderful base for a product for sensitive skin.

The list of available carriers is too long and detailed for this book. The only purpose of this list is to suggest that carriers are important to choosing a lotion according to the purpose to be addressed in its use. Information is the key to reading these labels, and, before choosing a product it is to the purchaser's advantage to look up the specific qualities of its ingredients.

Keep in mind that many times the combination of two ingredients will enhance their individual benefits for use and will be a fact that is normally unknown by us, the uneducated. For that reason, we must hope that the person on the 800 number at a product company will know enough to answer our questions. If not, ask for someone who does!

Essential Oils. Essential oils are available to us in lotions that are reliable and safe through the design of specialists called formulators and cosmetic chemists. The function of these oils in lotions is both therapeutic and aromatic. The results of spa manicures can change dramatically with the correct choice of aromatherapy lotion for clients. Information is the key to success in aromatherapy, too.

There are thousands of essential oils. If a professional is interested, study of essential oils is fascinating and informative. However, unless she is a cosmetic chemist or is sincerely interested in becoming an expert on these oils and willing to find and study the information, she

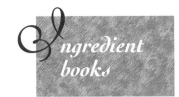

Ingredient books

The formulators of lotions will groan when reading that I suggest looking up the ingredients because sometimes the phrase "a little knowledge hurts" applies here. However, I feel we must know the basics of what we present to our clients, and this is where we can find that information, however basic it is. Also, some lotions are full of chemicals and provide no benefit to our clients other than "feeling good" at the moment of use. Clients of nail spas deserve better than this, and it is our responsibility to ferret out this information This is where we start.

must do as I do—use an aromatherapy book outlining their overall properties. This will provide basic knowledge of what is being purchased, if the nail spa wishes to use them in their oil form. (Call the company for specific questions.) Choose several that are safe, according to research, and produce the desired results, then test them for free on a willing volunteer. This method provides a considerable improvement over past uninformed product choices, and is clearly apparent in the effectiveness for clients.

Many spa manicurists who incorporate essential oils into their work chose one for calming and one for energizing. I suggest the spa stays basic in the choices unless the oils are studied in depth by the users. Many aromatherapy companies now provide information for their purchasers, enabling us to use them safely.

Lotion Purposes, According to the Ingredients

We become informed purchasers when we acquire sufficient information. Using the product label, the resource person can develop a balanced set of lotions to support the procedures at the table and to offer as home care. The five basic lotions that can be useful for skin care for the hands and feet are massage, moisturizing, sloughing, chemical exfoliating, and barrier lotions.

Massage Lotions. A massage lotion must have a quality often referred to as *slippage*. It must allow the spa manicurist to maintain smooth, liquid movements on the surface of the skin and minimize any drag. Another quality it must have is *hold*. This allows the hand, as it is slipping over the body, to remain against the skin, holding treatment ingredients against the surface in the massage movements.

Many professionals believe the ideal massage lotion does not absorb into the skin quickly, reducing the number of reapplications necessary to maintain a comfortable slip. For these professionals, the purpose of this lotion is only to provide this slippage and hold, not for offering nourishment and treatment properties.

Most massage lotions have similar basic ingredients. Many have a mineral oil base or list mineral oil as one of the first three ingredients. Others have glycerine or glycerol, spreading agents that help the hands move smoothly over the client's skin. Because mineral oil and glycerine have large molecules, most products with these ingredients will stay on the surface of the skin and produce a shiny, protective film. They usually have little lasting treatment value because they are not absorbed well, though they may have excellent barrier qualities.

Some massage lotions are designed not only to aid and enhance the massage but also to provide some therapeutic benefits, such as hydration and moisturization. Certain essential oils can be designed into the lotions as the carriers to provide these properties. Usually these lotions are more expensive and must be reapplied more often during the massage than the mineral oil-based lotions. (More product is used in the procedure.) Personally, I prefer my massage lotion to provide more than slippage, so I choose a lotion that also moisturizes the client's skin. (A moisturizing lotion with less slip/hold than the mineral oil-based products can still be used for the massage with the addition of more applications of the product.)

There are additional reasons I prefer the more therapeutic (and more expensive) lotion for massage. I intensely dislike the residual greasy feel of most traditional massage lotions and their influence on what I do next. I always resort to wiping my hands with a towel to proceed. I also believe my own hands are in better shape if I can use moisturizing lotions as much as possible in my work activities.

Moisturizing Lotions. Moisturizing lotions are more quickly absorbed. They produce obvious, long-lasting effects, and leave no greasy residue after absorption. When a good moisturizing lotion is applied, it produces an immediate improvement in the hands that is apparent to the client. Many of these lotions carry nutrients, such as vitamins and minerals, into the layers of the skin and apply antioxidants along with their moisturizers. Essential oils with tiny molecules are usually used to accomplish their purposes. (Fig. 11–3) Moisturizing lotions are extremely beneficial for dry, irritated skin and are the most widely sold lotions in our repertoire of home care lotions.

Sloughing (Mechanical Exfoliation) Lotions. A sloughing lotion mechanically removes the dead surface cells of the skin. Most contain an abrasive such as pumice, cornmeal, or ground apricot pits that make the lotion grainy. Others will contain beads that will slough the dead cells without excessively abrading the surface of the skin. (I personally prefer the less abrasive sloughers; I avoid products with pumice as an ingredient, for example, especially for clients who have chaffing.) The action of rubbing the abrasive against the skin removes the dead epithelial cells. As the professional massages the client's skin, some of the lotions dry into a rough granular paste that contains the dead cells and sloughing granules. (Fig. 11–4)

Some sloughing lotions also contain essential oils or vitamins to provide an additional benefit as the professional massages the product into the skin. It will always be necessary, though, to remove the residue left by the grainy sloughing lotions and to apply a good moisturizing lotion

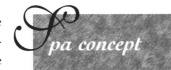

Jody Achatz, Salon Manager, Kenneth's Designgroup and Day Spa, Hilliard, OH

Before we incorporated spa manicuring into our nail spa, it was a very good nail room, but not a nail spa. The nail technicians were highly trained, and their work was top quality, but they did not do as well as the rest of the salon in income or retail or in comments from our clients. Most of all, they did not seem to feel like part of the salon or spa. They felt like step-children. We were searching for a way to change this situation. We feel we found this in the concept of being spa. We brought in an educator and upgraded the menu and the products. We focused on making this change, and it worked both for them and for us.

Since we educated the nail technicians into the concept of being spa, they have not only upgraded their skills, they have more than doubled their home care sales and their client retention has sky rocketed. They are knowledgeable and skilled, and it shows. Their room has changed in both atmosphere and name; we now proudly call it "The Nail Spa at Kenneth's" and added a beautiful glass door as entry. They are now called spa nail professionals, not nail technicians. They have become a cohesive and wonderfully pleasant group to work with in the salon and spa. Along with all of this, their service income has zoomed. All of us are happy! They only problem? They are overbooked and overworked, and we must hire more professionals. What a problem to have!

Figure 11-3

Many moisturizing lotions contain vitamins and minerals, which show immediate results to clients.

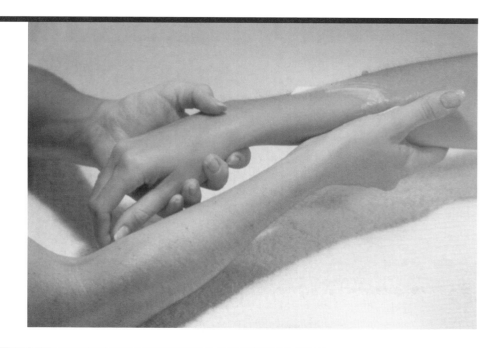

Figure 11-4

Sloughing lotion is abrasive, and removes dead surface cells of the skin.

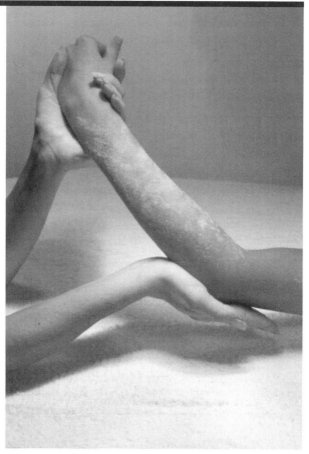

afterward. Some sloughers are available, however, that have granules that "melt" on the skin when lotion is applied. This saves the professional time and effort in the service.

Chemical Exfoliating Lotion. This lotion contains chemicals that facilitate the release of the outer layer of dead cells of the epithelium by dissolving their natural intercellular adhesive. This release of cells is called *desquamation*. Retaining this layer of dead cells emphasizes wrinkles and makes the skin appear older. Releasing the dead cells reveals fresh living tissue that is softer and younger looking.

The chemicals most often used in exfoliating lotions are alpha hydroxy acids (AHAs) derived from plants, such as sugar cane and apples, or other natural sources, such as milk or wine. (see Chapter 10). It is important to know certain facts about an exfoliating lotion; including the percentage of AHA, the pH, and the purity. This information is rarely placed on the label (see Chapter 10). However, we can discern some basics simply by reading the labels and interpreting the language. Not all formulations will fall into the following categories but most will.

- Lotions containing less than 5% AHAs are "just lotions," though improved moisturizers. Most drug store/department store lotions are these percentages to guard against lawsuits. Their labels will state "Alpha Hydroxy Acid," though not the percentage.

- Lotions containing 5% to 7% are sold by salons in prescriptive home care treatments for dry hands. They are highly effective moisturizing lotions and can be used very effectively in salon home care routines. Their labels say "apply generously several times per day" or something similar, and this will cause no irritation under usual circumstances.

- Lotions containing 7% to 9% AHAs are highly therapeutic and moisturizing. The labels may say "apply several times a day" and generally they will cause no irritation unless this is excessive. Some visible sloughing may occasionally occur if the higher percentage product is used excessively. Lotions with these percentages are not usually sold for general use for this reason. (If so, it is in salon retail to enable education.)

- Lotions over 9%, up to 15%, are sold as professional and medical home care exfoliation lotions for leathery, dry, and aging hands. Products for salon use are usually below 12%; physicians will sell up to 15% products. The labels of these products will say "apply one or twice daily," and mean it; overuse can cause irritation.

- Lotions of over 15% are mainly for *medical use only* and are generally used as a treatment for leathery and aging hands.

If a professional home care product restricts use to only once or twice a day, a purchaser can usually assume the AHA percentage is over 9%, likely 10% to 12%. Higher percentages than that should *never* be used as home care unless directed by a dermatologist, and it is definitely not recommended for use at all on clients with sensitive skin.

If a professional product claiming AHAs does not restrict its use in the directions, a purchaser can assume it contains enough AHA to be an excellent moisturizer but not enough to be an effective exfoliant. This lower percentage of AHA softens the intercellular adhesive enough to allow penetration of the lotion's emollient ingredients, but not enough to enhance natural exfoliation of the dead cells.

Introducing a client with dry skin to a good AHA lotion with either or both moisturizing and exfoliant properties can be the best treatment available. These lotions can dramatically improve the condition of the skin while perpetrating the effects of and enhancing a service's value in her view. However, if a client has any sensitivities, it might be best to stick to a good moisturizing lotion or combine its use with a low AHA lotion to be used only a few times per day. Professional gentle physical exfoliation will enhance the effects of the products.

Barrier Lotions. Under certain conditions, it is wise to recommend a client use a lotion with barrier qualities, meaning it will bar the dry heat or the cold from harming the skin, form a barrier to hold the skin's innate moisture inside, or hold in another lotion's ingredients. Mineral oil, the primary ingredient in many barrier lotions, has larger molecules that in most lotions only minimally or, at best, slowly absorb into the pores of the skin. (Mineral oil is a good moisturizer *if* it is absorbed.) The best philosophy is that a product with mineral oil listed in the first two or three ingredients will prevent the escape of natural oils and moisture and encourage the production of natural oils.

Barrier lotions have an important place in home care. Clients can be instructed to use a moisturizing lotion at bedtime and, once it has been absorbed, follow it with a barrier lotion to help the skin retain the nutrients and moisturizers they have applied previously.

Another important function of a barrier lotion is as a protectant against adverse environmental conditions, such as wind and sun, with the addition of SPFs, of course. A mineral oil with large molecules is an excellent carrier for these products due to its poor absorption. A third function is as a carrier for AHAs in high percentage AHA exfoliating lotions. In chemical exfoliating lotions, it is desirable to keep the AHAs on the surface of the skin for a time rather than having them absorbed, allowing them to do their job on the stratum corneum before moving to the lower levels of the epidermis.

A fourth use of mineral oil in lotions will be in a barrier lotion designed as a protectant against chemicals and irritants. These lotions must sit on the surface of the skin to serve as a protectant. The design challenge is to use the mineral oil in a way that will not produce a greasy feeling while maintaining the protectants on the surface of the skin only.

SPF Lotions

Until recently, hand care professionals have paid little attention to the prevention of ultraviolet (UV) ray damage to the skin. The spa manicurist must consider this an important aspect of her client recommendations, however. The sun's damage to the lower layers of the skin produces the ugly age spots that our clients detest, and SPF lotions are their only defense against them, other than staying completely out of the sun. (These rays can also cause skin cancer.)

A client who wishes to prevent or reduce the production of further age spots, or is using hydroquinone and exfoliating treatments to reduce them, *must* use an SPF lotion whenever she is exposed to the sun. That lotion should be an SPF 15, or above, to block the UV rays that damage the basal layer of the skin.

Choosing Lotions

Deciding which lotion each client needs is a skill that soon becomes second nature. Professionals learn it by developing analytical skills, examining lotion ingredient lists, and assessing the needs of their clients. Their job is to choose the lotions that best serve the clients' purposes and to avoid lotions with expensive or unnecessary ingredients. The products that work best for her and her clients are chosen after learning as much as possible about lotion ingredients, resourcing the best products, and experimenting with the different possible choices.

Many professionals avoid products that have an abundance of chemical-sounding names in their list of ingredients because some clients will make purchasing decisions by taking a look at the list. For that reason, many product companies are using the space on their ingredient lists to more fully explain the "chemicals," such as lists that include the familiar names Topopheral (Vitamin E) and Ascorbic Acid (Vitamin C) are examples.

Balancing a Nail Spa Lotion Menu

Balance in a lotion menu means resourcing only the lotions that meet one or more of the needs on the retail and professional menus and avoiding purchase of extra, overlapping lotions. Some will be both retail (R) and professional (P) preparations. These are the ones I suggest for a spa concept salon:

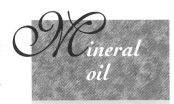

Mineral oil

This much maligned ingredient is available in grades, each more easily absorbed than the lesser refined grade. For that reason, cosmetic products can theoretically contain mineral oil that will absorb adequately for the purpose of moisturization. These absorbable products will be more expensive than those containing the lesser refined grade of mineral oil. How do we tell which grade of mineral oil is in a product prior to purchase? There is no way to know for sure.

Personally, when I am checking or purchasing products, I avoid lotions that have mineral oil because of this problem. The exception is when I am purchasing a barrier lotion or a lotion designed to carry AHA to the skin.

Many formulators avoid the use of even the highly refined mineral oil for moisturization because of its reputation. This reputation was earned by the use of poorer grades of mineral oil by formulators in cosmetic products in prior times. The resulting reputation will take many years to correct, if it ever happens. In the meantime, I avoid products that have mineral oil in their list of ingredients because I have no way of knowing what grade is being used.

- A "low" AHA lotion for moisturizing/hydration of dry hands (R)

  This product is an excellent professional retail item.

- A lotion for intense hydration (R/P)

  This product is used in several manicures as a moisturizer/hydrator, and for sensitive and dry skin in retail. It may be an aromatherapy lotion, also.

- A high percentage AHA for dry, leathery skin (R/P)

  This product is retailed for use once or twice a day for dry, leathery skin and aging, and for discolored skin. It is a treatment lotion used only during professional services and as directed in home care.

- An aromatherapy or mineral oil-based massage lotion (personal choice) (P)

  This is a heavier lotion for use during the massage.

- An SPF 15 lotion to block the ultraviolet ray damage of the basal layer of the skin (R)

  This product is applied every time the client will be exposed to the sun. (If the moisturizing lotion has SPF 15 ingredients, this lotion will be unnecessary.)

As increased knowledge about lotions is put into practice, a nail spa is certain to enhance its ability to meet client needs and increase the value of the services to them. The long-term results will be a higher income and a more loyal clientele.

CUTICLE TREATMENTS

Products for cuticle treatment in the past were usually cuticle solvents. We spent as little as possible on the one that was the most convenient to use. We used them to soften or dissolve the cuticles during a manicure and gave them little thought. They were strictly utilitarian and definitely not products that improved the condition of the client's cuticles. Rarely did we sell them as retail products.

Then, aromatherapy cuticle treatments were introduced. They did not change our services too much—we still wanted that solvent on those cuticles to soften them—but we routinely sold the aromatherapy oils for home use because they conditioned the touch cuticle well. They became a staple on our retail shelf.

Then products came on the market that really made the difference: cuticle lotions and creams containing AHAs. This is the ultimate (thus far) product for cuticle home care. They make life much easier for the client with leather cuticles and for her manicurist who must deal with them! Nail spas should find, test, and choose AHA home care cuticle treatments for their clients. They will see a dramatic difference with this addition to their treatment because it exfoliates the dead cells from the client's cuticles. These products are especially good when used in tandem with aromatherapy cuticle oils, which soften and nourish the cuticles.

A new cuticle treatment is now available that focuses on destroying bacteria, fungi, and viruses while softening the cuticles. These products are designed for use on clients with torn, abused cuticles and especially for their use at home. With the new focus on sanitation and treatment products, these are good products for home care and for use professionally on clients with torn cuticles. They can also be sent home with the client when a spa manicurist accidentally nicks her.

Cuticle Oils

Cuticle oils can be used to soften cuticles during spa treatments and before application of AHA cuticle treatments in the home care regimen, especially if a matrix massage is in the client's home care regimen. The oils should be chosen for their nutrient and moisturizing properties and for their ability to penetrate within seconds, leaving no oily residue. The client should be educated on how to massage in the product daily to stimulate the matrix and moisturize the cuticles around the nails.

NAIL HARDENERS AND TREATMENTS

Nail hardeners and treatments are an essential part of the treatment and home care tools for the spa manicurist. They have been an important part of the new successes of the manicuring industry. They should be used responsibly and with full knowledge of the conditions of the nails. They are discussed in Chapter 2.

TOP COATS AND BASE COATS

Top coats and base coats of the past had little to offer except retention for the base coats and gloss for the top coats. Clients were forced to spend up to an hour lounging in the nail salon waiting for their polish

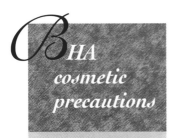
BHA cosmetic precautions

Precautions to be noted in recommending BHA cosmetics for a client are its potentials for irritations and allergies. Although BHA products will not cause any problems for the majority of clients; those with cosmetically sensitive skin should be use tested, meaning the product should be used on a small area exactly in the recommended regimen for a few days or even a few weeks before widening its scope to the full area of use.

Clients who are prone to allergies should have a cosmetic patch test for sensitivity. If no reaction is noted, the client can assume she is not sensitive to BHA.

Clients who have allergies to aspirin or other salicylates should not use cosmetics containing BHAs. Cosmetic products with salicylic ingredients will typically be sunscreens, acne treatments, and exfoliates.

to dry if they wished their polish to be perfect. Then the fast-drying top coats appeared, and both clients and the nail technicians were thrilled! We could polish them and they could be out the door within minutes, without that inevitable return for correcting a smudge.

We now have wide choices of top coats and base coats, with newer ones coming out every day. These choices support one of the aspects of spa that I recommend: the nail services in a nail spa should have a drying routine that is better than just ushering the client out the door with her hands in the air. The routine should be a relaxing few minutes, after the service, that ensures the nails are completely dry before the client leaves. A refreshment, reading material, and a comfortable chair should be offered, whether it is at an available nail table or in the lobby, after her reappointment. Optimally, the client is moved from the service table.

Following are some suggestions for choosing and applying the post-service products for natural nails:

1. Use base coats as base coats, top coats as top coats. Base coats are stickier to the touch and have no gloss. Top coats will be glossy and tend to peel from the nail plate when directly applied to them; polish will not adhere to them well.

2. Choose a base coat and top coat *system*, not products from different lines. Products have different drying times and application techniques. If they are not compatible, the polish may peel or bubble. (An exception may be when a treatment product is used.)

3. Choose a base coat that works well on natural nails. (Usually this one will work well on acrylics also, but not always the reverse.) This search can be a chore because many are designed to work best on acrylics. However, because natural nails are becoming popular again, many base coats are coming on the market that will serve this clientele well.

4. The chosen product should be compatible with the way the professionals apply their products or they will need to be retrained to meet the products' needs. Does the base coat have to be dry before adding the polishes? Does the polish have to be dry or wet before the top coat is applied? Many products have specific technique needs if the polish is to be durable and beautiful. Read the directions.

5. The top coat chosen to be a home care product may have to be different than the one used in the salon. A top coat that the professionals use because it goes on well over wet

polish will not work for the client who is adding it over dry polish for renewal of a gloss at home. It may peel. Resourcing top coats for their specific purpose is important to their success.

6. Add thinner to a top coat product that has thickened over time. A thick top coat is difficult to apply and will streak.

7. Always purchase a thinner from the same company as the top coat. The chemistry of a product may be a unique mixture of ingredients that may need to be maintained in its thinner. Further, acetone should not be used for thinning these products because it quickly breaks down the chemistry.

8. Purchase a product that claims to be non-yellowing and train the clients about maintaining this property, according to manufacturer directions. If there are repeated complaints, change to another product.

9. Train every new manicurist in perfect polish application. No matter how wonderful the client's service is, she will judge the perfection on the appearance of the polish.

10. Encourage the client to renew the polish by applying a quality top coat every 2 to 3 days.

ACCESSORY PRODUCTS: FILLING IN THE BLANKS

Many salons will sell accessory products to fill other needs of their clients. These products should have one or all of the following properties:

- They should be available only in salons. (professional only).
- They should be of higher quality than is available outside the salon or in non-professional beauty supply stores.
- They should meet a special need for a special client.

Latex or nonlatex gloves can be sold to encourage their use in the client's daily activities. They should be good gloves (they can purchase the junk ones at the grocery), which the nail spa can purchase at the medical or dental supply in bulk, or sources can be researched in the industry. Accompany them with cotton glove liners, which can also be purchased in packages of 12 pairs. The two products can be packaged together in a plastic bag, with a computer-generated label slipped inside to show the contents, size, and price. Enough can be charged to make the effort more than worth it, and the clients like the convenience. When the spa manicurist sees during an analysis that a client needs them (most everyone), she can lay them on the table beside the client and strongly suggest their use. The clients become addicted to

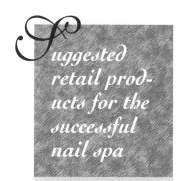

the quality of the gloves and the absorption of perspiration by the glove liners and repurchases the packet often. (Some salons even package the outer gloves separately.)

Another accessory item is a ceramic file that shapes and seals a client's natural nail instead of abrading it, causing layering. Clients like it because it is easy to use; manicurists like it because it is nonagressive in home care.

I suggest that nail spas routinely audit their shelves. Those products that have been taking up space (and holding money hostage) for more than 2 months should be re-evaluated for their productivity to the inventory list. If they are worthwhile to keep, the spa professionals should be retrained for their use and benefits to the clients. If they are not worthwhile, they should be placed on "special" and taken off the inventory list. The salon cannot afford non-productive shelf space. (Fig. 11–5)

TRAINING PROFESSIONALS FOR RETAIL

Training in retailing and product knowledge is the final preparation toward achieving retail success in a nail spa. It is a major part of preparation for the spa and professional's success with new manicures and products, and for growth of the clientele. The sequence goes like this:

- A nail spa resources, tests, and purchases a balanced retail inventory that supports the service menu.

- The spa manicurist is trained in how the products are used at the table and in home care.

- She is trained in how to partner with the client in professional and home care for perpetuating the results of her services.

- An attractive display is designed and placed within easy access of the professional and client.

- She "trains" her clients in home care.

- The clients sense the knowledge of the professional and are willing to purchase the product; they'll try it "just this once." Because of her needs-targeted training by the spa manicurist, she does her home care.

- The professional service is perpetuated, through the home care. The client sees positive results and is impressed! She is going to continue these services and listen to "her spa manicurist." She will follow the spa manicurist's future recommendations for home care products and services.

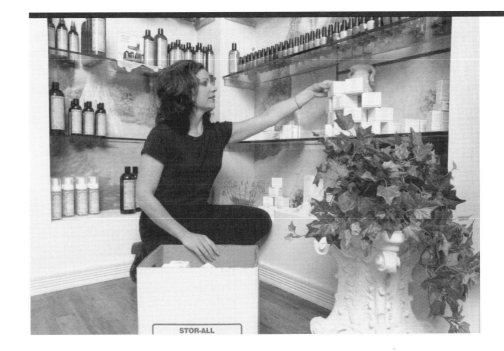

Figure 11-5

Nail spa professionals
must know the ingredients
of products their and
benefits to be able to
educate their clients.

- The spa manicurist's client list, as well as the nail spa's, is growing because she is having great results on her clients.
- Her clients are recommending the nail spa and the spa manicurist to their friends.
- The amount of home care products sold is skyrocketing. The spa manicurist's income takes a big leap!
- The nail spa's income is skyrocketing. The percentage of retail to income is higher than it ever has been and growing.
- Now, everyone is happy—the client, the professional, the management, and the owner!

We know that not all clients will purchase home care products right after their service, some never will. This does not alleviate the technician's responsibility to make suggestions, and explain the benefits of home care products. If the client doesn't receive and understand this information, all the aforementioned benefits are cancelled and the visit looses its therapeutic effects. It is no longer spa concept.

WHAT TO SELL, WHEN

One of the home care issues for a spa manicurist is "what to sell, when." With the appropriate education and available products, these professionals will develop a sense for this key aspect of retailing. For instance, a client whose skin is very dry may have dry cuticles and weak, possibly peeling, nails. What is recommended to this client first? If the spa manicurist attempts to send her home with all her product needs she may become overwhelmed and discouraged.

This client needs to go home with her nail treatment and her cuticle oil first, but the manicurist must also mention her future needs. While showing her how to use the products, say, "The oil will soften your cuticles and the treatment will get your nails started toward hardening. Next week we will do a gentle exfoliation and hydration of your skin and get you started on the appropriate lotions for your skin. You're going to have new hands and great nails in no time. Let's set up that appointment right now." The client will walk out with products that will give her an immediate change in her nails and cuticles, with her assignment and an appointment. She knows that next week she will learn how to improve her skin and will take home skin care products.

The balance and design of the retail list and full training of professionals to promote the products can produce higher profits, a longer client list, and more income for the professionals. It takes research and work on an ongoing basis, but it is rewarding for everyone and builds enthusiasm, from the client to the owner.

First Impressions Count

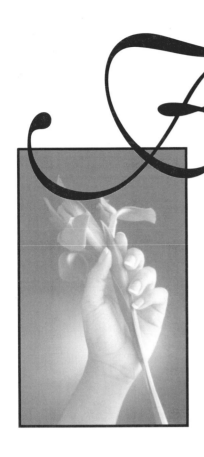

12

OBJECTIVES

At the end of this chapter, you should be able to:

- Design a spa concept entrance routine for clients.
- Design entry written materials for use by the clients.
- Design a client information questionnaire.
- State the reasons for collecting client information.

Preservice details are an integral part of professional service in a salon and are especially important in spa concept. The client's connection with the overall salon, spa, or nail spa, the professional, and the services provided begins when she enters and likely sets the tone for her visit. Her first impression must support a positive experience.

CLIENT ENTRANCE

Most new clients will consciously or unconsciously check out a salon when they first enter the lobby. They want to have a positive experience and it is up to the staff to provide them a reason to gladly return. The following details are essential for providing the support new clients need for them to want to return.

Receptionist. A receptionist must be friendly, maintain a genuine smile and make eye contact with the client. (This person *must* like people.) (Fig. 12–1) Eye contact by the receptionist introduces a feeling of inclusive and exclusive attentiveness by the salon, a feeling the client wants to feel when she first enters. The receptionist in a successful nail spa will verbally welcome her, use her name when addressing her and answer her questions completely, before they are asked, if possible. A good receptionist knows what the clients will want to ask and be eager to provide the answers. This supports the client's immediate feeling of being number one in the eyes of the nail spa.

A receptionist, or someone designated to that responsibility, is responsible for beginning the pampering procedures. Some salons and day

Figure 12-1

A receptionist must enjoy people so that she can perform her job well.

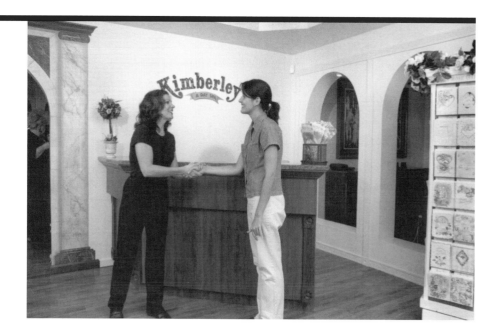

Spa Manicuring for the Salon and Spa

spas have salon coordinators who share this responsibility with the receptionist. No client likes to haul her coat around, observe a mess, or try to locate where she is supposed to be.

The receptionist is the first and last contact clients have with a salon and the person clients may remember most as representative of the salon or nail spa's philosophy toward them. Clients willingly give their hard earned money to a salon whose receptionist they believe cares about their comfort, but not to one whose receptionist is rudeness personified. This person may be given only one chance, and so may the salon.

A salon with no receptionist can succeed in this area, also, sometimes more easily than the larger salon. The separation of the professional from the entering clients in a large salon or spa highly accentuates the importance of introducing the client correctly from the front desk to the nail spa and professional. In a small nail spa with no receptionist where the professional has this responsibility, the client can quickly connect to her professional and the nail spa if the introduction and entry are done correctly. All these introductory procedures are the professional's responsibility; no short cuts should be taken.

It should be mentioned here that when a nail spa is too busy for the professionals to do the entry procedures correctly, it may be time for the owner to consider hiring a receptionist. When receptionists are trained correctly and their responsibilities are well defined, they will easily pay for themselves by their presence.

Waiting Room Area. The waiting room must be *immaculate*, *neat*, and *welcoming*. (Fig. 12–2) Someone has to be responsible for the ongoing condition of the waiting areas; a beginning and end of the day straightening will not be enough. The condition of the area must support positive feelings the clients want to have right from the beginning of their visit, such as "This salon cares about me," "This salon is clean," "This salon is organized," and "This spa wants me here." Conversely, a messy waiting area may introduce opposite concepts and support any negative incidents or observations that might happen during the service.

Information. Introductory information should be given to the client in the waiting room and verbally explained by the receptionist in a pleasant and friendly tone. Clients hate to ask questions about forms. (Fig. 12–3) It makes them feel stupid. The introductory handouts should be as follows:

- Brief *policy information* should be in written form enabling every client to understand, right from the first appointment, the nail spa's expectations of its clients. Clients have expectations and need to know what the nail spa's are, also.

Figure 12-2

The waiting room provides a pleasant impression for the entering client.

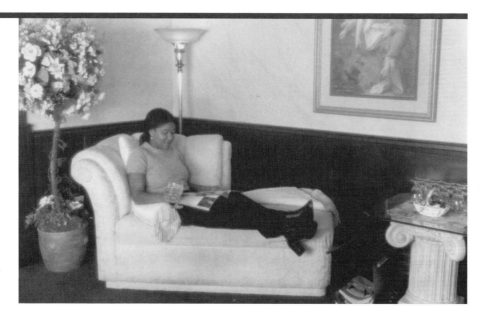

Figure 12-3

Written information is explained by a friendly receptionist.

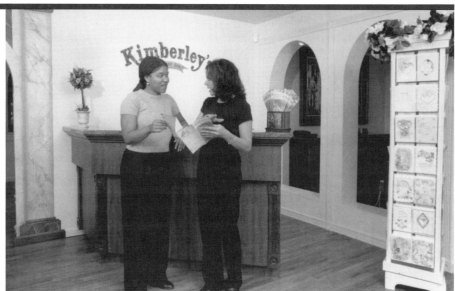

- A *client information card* and pen/pencil should be included in new client information. These records should be filled out by the client, then used by the spa manicurist during the client analysis. Appoint a new client 15 minutes early to give them ample time.
- A *service menu*, a list of the nail spa's service offerings, should be included to enable the client to know what experiences are available. The services should be described briefly as part of the list.
- A *price list*, a listing of the nail spa's services followed by the prices, will be a separate sheet included in the service menu. (Fig. 12–4)

These may or may not be in separate pieces and should be concise; clients are more comfortable with less to carry than more. When these are all in one handout, it's a *brochure.*

Client Transfer. The transfer of the client to the nail table should be a comfortable and welcoming routine by a person responsible for the transition, a receptionist, a spa coordinator, or the spa manicure professional. A client who must wander around to find the spa manicurist she is assigned to will feel neglected and be ready to note other negative details. For the first visit, an introduction to the nail professional by the transition person, or by the professional herself, is also important, with a friendly "hello" and a mention of the professional's name, the client's name, and the service. ("Hello, Ms. Jones. My name is Jane, and I'm going to do your manicure today. Please come with me/Please have a seat.") Throughout the service, the client's name should be used several times. (Fig. 12–5)

Punctuality. A punctual professional is important in a nail spa, especially when the client is new. However, if the professional is running late, a smiling receptionist or fellow professional should make the client comfortable at a clean and clear station, offer her a refreshment, and offer a placating service, such as placing her hands in warm mitts.

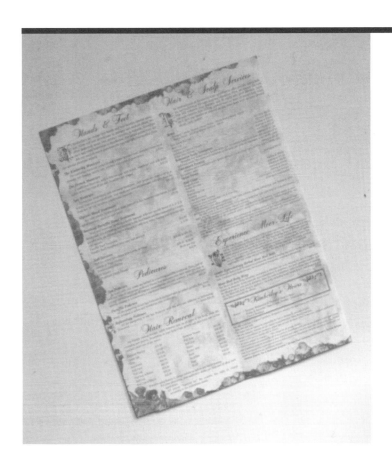

Figure 12-4

Placing prices on a separate sheet will allow changes without forcing the printing of a new brochure.

Figure 12-5

Introduction of a client to her professional suggests that her comfort is important to the spa.

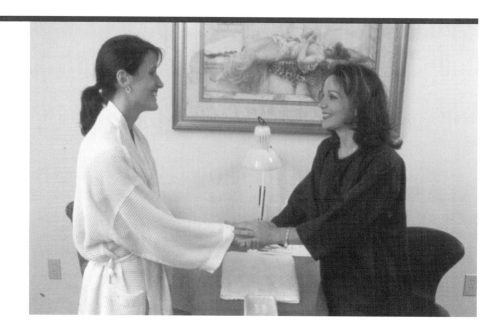

It is important to have the clients seated at the appointed time. Many salons purposely have that extra, clean, unmanned station for use during those times of running late, accidental overbookings, and other emergencies. If this is impossible, the details of designing comforting techniques and policies for handling these situations are essential to maintaining spa concept.

Repeat Client Entrance

The salon entrance routine for the repeat client is little different from that of the new client, except that there is no information to read nor questions to answer. However, she still has the same expectations for a bright, clean, and straightened waiting room and for a friendly receptionist and spa manicurist. She performs the scrub routine before sitting down at the table. The professional is responsible for perusing her client records—her services, home care, health and so on. She may ask the client if there have been any changes in her address and telephone and may ask the appropriate questions about any health care changes that may have occurred since her last visit. (This is dictated by their familiarity, of course.)

Entrance routines show professionalism and a caring attitude and are a part of spa concept. They are a significant part of the success of a nail spa.

WRITTEN MATERIALS

The written materials provided the new client should fit the ambiance of the overall salon. For instance, a client will expect a glossy and beautifully printer-designed set of information that coordinates with the interior ambiance from a large upscale salon or day spa with expensive decor. Inconsistent materials will be noticed immediately as something out of place. Conversely, a small nails-only salon, though it may be fully spa concept, is not expected to have glossy, fancy materials; actually, the client may feel such materials are overly pretentious and expensive. She may be thinking, "The prices are going to be very high here." Attractive computer-generated materials may be more appropriate.

The materials, whatever the cost, should be well integrated: they should cover the needed information and fit together, possibly inside the largest piece or in a packet, or all in a brochure, except the client card. This prevents paper shuffling by the client and fostering a temptation to drop it all into the nearest trash can. A well-done set of materials will be seen as a positive representation of the information the client wants to know about the salon, spa, or nail spa. A poorly done set will be seen as "junk mail," something to dispose of as quickly as possible.

Salon Policies. Clients get to know the salon, spa or nail spa through a list of policies that support the activities within spa concept and allow the business procedures to run smoothly. The policies should be written in an attractive, friendly but formal "welcome" format and handed to her, printed on or placed separately inside the other materials, along with a refreshment.

Policies must be well thought out and kept as brief as possible. They should be worded carefully to avoid seeming like "rules" even though that is what they are. The salon's name and telephone number should be evident, of course, and the first sentence should welcome the client to the salon. The remaining contents are different for each nail spa. The designer might visit several other salons and note what they have included in their new client information before writing her own. Examples of contents could be:

1. A statement of what the salon's goals will be for the client's visit, such as, "We, at XX Salon, want to provide you with a relaxing visit in which we will relax, beautify and rejuvenate…"

2. A reappointment policy, such as, "To ensure that you will be able to visit our salon again at a convenient time to you, we suggest that you make your next appointment prior to your leaving the salon today."

3. A no-show policy, such as, "We are happy to reserve time for your next visit at a time convenient to you. However, when you fail to cancel, you prevent another client from using that time and render the professional to be inactive.

We ask that…" Many owners choose not to include this policy because they feel it generates a negative aspect. The policy designer will make this decision.

4. A smoking policy should be stated for both smokers and nonsmokers to see, such as, "Our city has designated our salon a "clean air environment…" (Pass the buck if you can, here.) Or, "For the comfort of our clients, we have an area designated for smoking…." Some clients may define where they spend their money next time on this issue.

5. A nail repair policy, such as, "We understand that the need for periodic nail repairs are inevitable. To accommodate you…"

6. A sanitation statement, such as, "Because we care…" (see Chapter 13). Possibly, it can be displayed to ensure its notice, but it should also be stated clearly in your client information.

7. A policy statement concerning children in the salon. Everyone has an opinion on this one. The policy maker must consider whether the presence of children is spa concept, whether they may deny others their spa experience. If it is a policy of exclusion, it must be stated in the written material clearly and carefully so mothers cannot claim they did not see it.

Policy information pieces should fit neatly inside the service menu, if they are separate, to keep paper shuffling to a minimum. An alternative is placing the salon policies on the back of the service menu, if space allows, keeping them brief and low key. Salons that have been in business for many years will have few changes in their policies, will change their services less often, and prefer to place their policies on their menu. This is advantageous because clients will see them every time they are given a list of services to inspect.

Policy information should reflect a caring, professional demeanor and can be signed by the owner for a personal and softening touch.

Service Menu

The service menu is an attractive listing of the services. The listing should include a detailed description of all the services to enable the client to understand exactly what will be experienced during the service. It uses language that entices a reader to appoint.

Manicure services should be described in detail similar to the other services. Describing the hair and facial services fully, then listing the services in the nail spa as "manicures and pedicures" will dramatically lower the traffic in the department by indicating that the salon perceives them at a diminished value.

The service menu may not show prices in it in spa concept salons and spas. However, it will usually be the largest piece of written information for the new client and other marketing materials can be included. These may include the salon's service philosophy, a biography of the owner, and more if it fits in the ambiance. If these materials are included, the service menu becomes a brochure and will have additional uses in the marketing plan.

Price List

The price list is an important part of entrance materials. New clients like to see this information in print and may tuck it away for future use or share it with friends. Existing clients like to be able to see the prices in print also so they do not have to ask what they are.

As with the rest of the printed materials, a formal price list should fit the ambiance and the budget. It can be a commercial printer-generated glossy or a well-designed computer-generated one. Clients would expect a large and luxurious nail spa to have a commercially designed and printed price list, though they would not expect it of a single technician in a lease station or small studio.

A separate price list is a simple list of the services and their prices without any service descriptions. It should fit inside the dominant piece of information provided the client, which is usually the service menu or the larger brochure.

A separate price list can be easily changed without harming the other marketing pieces. Consider this, I was in a beautiful spa and picked up a nicely done, commercially designed and printed brochure. I opened it to have a look and found the prices were marked out with white out and written over with a pen. The new client may see this spa's attitudes toward her as "you aren't worth the effort, even when you first visit us." At least it casts an image of messiness, which can carry over to a general feeling about the overall spa. This spa should have had either computer-generated materials that could have been easily changed, placed the price sheet inside as an insert, or waited for new materials to be printed before changing the prices.

The marked over service menu/price sheet occurs often and is unacceptable in spa concept salons. The introductory information must present an attractive beginning to every new client. For many spas that means separate price lists that can be inserted into the service menu unless the segment on which it is contained can be reprinted quickly, easily, and inexpensively.

Formatting the Information

Modern technology has made computer-generated salon information acceptable for some salons if the design is well done and the paper is high quality. Computer programs are available now that are quite user-friendly and provide templates (predesigned patterns) that will result in a beautiful presentation.

The least expensive way, of course, is for the owner, if he or she has the patience, an employee who has the capability, or a computer-addicted friend to do the designing. If not, having a computer design specialist design it after the owner decides on the format and information is still less expensive than contracting for printer-generated paperwork from a printer. Computer-generated materials can be maintained and changed when the need arises, copied in manageable numbers at the local copy shop, and quickly available when more are needed. The disk will be held by the nail spa for any later minor changes. (The nail spa keeps it, not the computer designer.)

Another issue for client introductory materials is the frequency with which it should be changed. Many marketing specialists will tell owners that it is important to change their printed client materials periodically to provide a "fresh look" to the salon (without redecorating!), and to announce and explain new services when they are added.

When the materials are redesigned, a whole new look should be achieved, and the new set immediately handed out to existing clients. Loyal clients want to be the first to know what is happening in 'their' salons and are the first to respond by booking appointments for new services. The new materials are handed to them with their next appointment card. This will give them a reminder of the salon's services, highlight the spa's client orientation, and introduce new services to them in printed form. Current clients see new materials as a sign the salon is doing well, and they like to be in a part of a successful salon or spa.

CLIENT RECORDS

When the new client enters, she should be provided with a questionnaire to record full information concerning her past services, her medical history, her address and telephone, and her referral. (Fig. 12–6.) This client record can be a general card or one specific to each service, such as one for manicures and one for pedicures.

In most nail spas, the client records her information before the appointment. However, in some the first professional she meets may do it for her as part of the analysis step for new clients. These salons feel

Spa Manicuring for the Salon and Spa

it is important to do this for their clients. The receptionist may fill in the client's name, address, telephone number, and referral information to save time used during the analysis. This information is collected during the telephone call when she makes her appointment.

The questions and design of client records vary according to the needs of the spa and the skills. They may be a 4"x 6" card that fits in a standard container or a 8-1/2"x 11" sheet. They may fit in a card box or in a ring binder, or whatever is the choice of management. Each nail spa will choose one that fits its needs. Generic ones are available for purchase.

If you do acrylics in the salon, questions relevant to their application can be on the back of the general card. If so, a line, such as, *"Please fill out the back of the card for an acrylic service,"* must be added, and the signature line moved to the back. The service grid can be below this. A few sample questions would be:

Have you worn nail enhancements prior to this time? _____
If so, what kind?_____
Are you allergic to any kind of enhancement? _____
If so, what kind? _____
Is your skin oily or dry? _____

Reasons for Client Records

Many salons and spas do not use client records. In a recent trade magazine, a professional said her boss did not allow her to use the information because she did not want them available to take if "someone" would leave. How naive! If that professional wants the information, she will get it, whether it is on paper or not. The logical reasons for collecting this information are:

- *Medical history of past physical disorders, causes and symptoms* — The manicurist must know what services are safe to recommend or not recommend.

- *Allergies and medications* — The presence of contraindications is important information. Some treatments cannot be recommended in the presence of certain allergies and medications, and taking risks is foolish. For example, clients using Retin A, a medication for acne conditions, should not have alpha hydroxy acids used on them unless their physician is contacted.

- *Prior treatments/tenderness* — Notations of problems with prior treatments are important to the treating professional. For example, a client who has arthritis may need a gentle touch

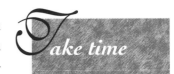

Take time

A wise owner will spend extended time developing the language and content of the salon introductory material. Diligent predesign will dramatically reduce the need for corrections and redesign. It especially results in saving money with commercially designed and printed materials. The more time they spend on your work, the more they charge; multiple edits will be a financial shock to an owner.

All computer-generated materials should be done on good paper stock that provides an attractive background. Thirty-eight pound paper is a good weight for a brochure, though more expensive, but it must be machine folded to achieve a finished look.

When in the design stages, ask for the opinions of others and redo the design until it is what you want and your reviewers agree is appropriate. These pieces of paper are the third impression of professionalism new clients have, immediately following the condition of the waiting room and the presentation by the receptionist.

Figure 12-6

General Preservice
Information Card.

Welcome to (Salon name)   (Please Print)

Name _____

Phone R _____ W _____

Address _____

City & Zip _____

Referred _____

Date _____

So that we may perform a quality service, please answer the following questions:

1. Occupation _____

2. Hobbies _____

3. Are you abusive to your hands? ___

    Do you wear gloves when cleaning? ___

4. Are your hands overly dry? ___ If yes, how do you treat this?

    _____

5. Do you have any allergies? ___

    If so, to what? _____

6. *Your health can be important to our professional care of your hands. Please circle any of the following that are relevant to your health, and fill in the name where necessary.*

Circulatory disease _____	Diabetes _____	Thyroid disorder _____
Heart disease _____	Skin diseases _____	Pregnancy _____
Acute arthritis _____	Lupus _____	Retin A therapy _____
Reynaud's disease _____	Fungal infection (hands or feet) _____	
Presently taking chemo/radiation _____	Using alpha hydroxy acids _____	

7. Are you currently on any medication on a regular basis? _____

    If so, what? _____

    Why? _____

8. Have you read and do you understand the information sheet provided you? _____

9. I have provided all relevant information for safe treatment.

Client's signature: _____

Technician: _____

on her knuckles. Knowledge of her tenderness will avoid pain and discomfort to the client and the necessity of telling the professional during each visit.

- *Prescribed treatments* — The manicurist must know what she has recommended in the past for the client, what works and does not work, and what she previously recommended for future treatments and manicures. Ignorance of these facts can cause mistreatment, and embarrassment, such as, "You told me xxx my last visit…"

- *Product sales* — The technician must know the products she has previously sold the client, so she will know what to recommend next, can check for improvement, and can avoid the aforementioned embarrassment. "You already sold that to me and I'm using it. Can't you tell?" We've all had it happen!

- *Legal protection* — A client who has not informed her spa professional of a problem cannot claim she has if she neglected to put the information in her record. These records are for the nail spa's and professional's protection. An example disclaimer, with the statement, "I have provided all relevant information for my nail professional" and requests a signature, will encourage the client to provide the pertinent information. (Although I do not claim to know all the potential pitfalls, these suggestions will provide information a spa can take to an attorney. A quick, advisory visit on salon issues, in general, can save the salon problems in the future.)

The owner who resists collection of these data is jeopardizing client safety, as well as the salon's and nail professional's continued ability to safely serve the client. It also provides some protection for the salon and professional from liability. We now live in a sue-happy society and must safeguard ourselves and our businesses from these liabilities in every way we can.

Service Grid

A service grid can be printed on the back of the card for noting service information, by date, and can provide space for the service professional to record additional information (see the client card), including home care products she has purchased, recommendations that have been made, and conditions that should be noted. These lines can act as personal marketing tools, also. Clients love for their nail professional to remember important events in their life. This information can be placed in her file here on the grid so the technician will be reminded to ask her about a recent special event the next time she comes in. It makes the nail professional look good, and the client feels special.

A unique form of shorthand can be developed by a professional for use on the grid. There are two reasons to do this: first, to provide quick information while allowing confidentiality, and second, to conserve space. I developed a shorthand of my own over my working years, such as "T" meant "trip" so I would write >T/HongKong/2w. The arrow meant that after her last appointment she went to Hong Kong for 2 weeks. Or >T/C/C1w, would mean that after that appointment she took a cruise in the Caribbean for 1 week. "TL" meant she talks loud. "Tch/CS," meant she was a teacher in the city schools. "N/Mem/IC" meant she was a nurse in Memorial Hospital Intensive Care Unit. "B/P" was important and does not mean British Petroleum. We all know what the B stands for, the P meant she was picky, too.

When designing the shorthand, always consider that the client may see the information accidentally or on purpose. (I had one take her card right out of my hand.) If shorthand cues are routinely written by the professional, she should be certain the cards are placed where the client cannot read them. I keep them inside my cabinet. I make the shorthand signals as difficult to interpret as possible, and place *nothing* in big red letters because it is usually assumed to be a negative statement by the observer.

A spa professional who uses her client information cards to their full potential will recognize them as one of her most valuable client relations tools. Their uses are limited only to the nail professional's desire for information. Other uses than the ones already mentioned are:

- *Personal idiosyncrasies* — A spa professional must be careful not to repeatedly suggest, discuss, or perform an act that is particularly annoying to a client (such as is the client with tender knuckles.)

- *Personal tenderness* — Some subjects will bring an emotionally upset client to tears. For instance, a valued client lost a child and reacted with tears when children were discussed in her presence. I wrote it down. Why cause her pain? These notations can provide information that can remind us of needed tender care for a client, at least until we know the client well enough to do without the reminders.

- *Controversial subjects* — Sometimes a professional must be reminded on client cards of subjects to avoid. One of my clients was an adamant supporter of a pyramid cosmetic company and would sit at my table and loudly and descriptively address the subject toward the general salon. Others will purposely discuss controversial subjects, such as religion and politics, to get the salon going. A professional can be better prepared with methods to keep these subjects from coming up, if there is information on the client's care to remind her.

Computer-Generated Client Records

If the salon or spa is computerized, client information may be permanently stored for printing out before each client visit, and a client information screen will be filled out by the spa manicurist after the service to note new conditions of importance. (Fig. 12–6)

Some computer systems will allow permanent storage of the information but will require the nail professional to pull it up before each visit for a visual check. This is a service responsibility of the spa professional. These systems require the professionals to pull up data twice in the day, once before the appointment and once for entering the data after the appointment. Other systems will provide a printout of all pertinent information for each client of the day, including past appointments, purchases, products and much more.

One issue of concern is that information in a computer system is too available to others, such as receptionists and other service providers. For this reason, delicate information about a client should be coded when recorded, as discussed above for a card system if you feel it should be kept confidential or is sensitive information. Allowing the broadcast of personal information about a client is ethically taboo, unprofessional and *very unwise.*

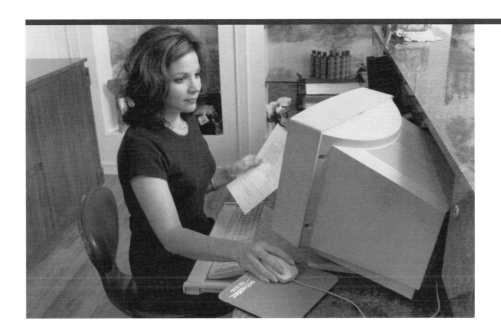

Figure 12-6

Client information can be permanently stored for output prior to each visit.

Client records are a "maintenance" duty and a wealth of information for the professional's use. Any situation, product, treatment, and so forth *must* be listed in the records to ensure effectiveness. Their maintenance is a discipline that must be incorporated quickly into the spa professional's service routine, a commitment of about 30 seconds per client.

This list of preservice salon introductory information is "basic," and many salons will add other materials for the new clients beyond this list, perhaps a product list, welcoming coupons, or event announcements. Every salon, spa, or nail spa will have its own personalized set of preservice materials, limited only by its own ideas and the needs of the clients and nail spa. The only requirement is that they should "fit" the ambiance and should be carefully integrated into the overall presentation of the materials to prevent the "junk mail" syndrome.

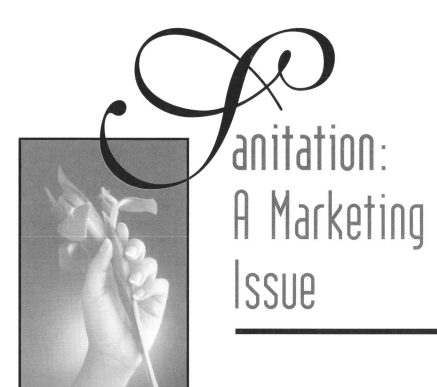

Sanitation: A Marketing Issue

13

OBJECTIVES

At the end of this chapter, you should be able to:

- State five ways to use sanitation as a marketing tool.
- Routinely inform the clients of sanitation procedures.
- Perform obvious sanitation for marketing as well as for protection purposes.
- Design a sign to inform the clients the spa uses high-level sanitation practices.
- Describe how the preservice scrub affects the profits of a salon or spa.
- Demonstrate the preservice scrub to a client.
- Perform basic implement sanitation.
- Establish/reinforce basic sanitation as a habit inside the table routine.

Nail professionals and spa manicurists constantly strive for professionalism and quality in their career and performance. However, as in any industry, a few "bad apples" have drawn negative press to our industry by the media calling attention to unsanitary salons. The poor sanitation habits in these targeted salons are great fuel for local TV stations and national "TV magazines" during sweeps months. These exposes bring reactions and much discussion from the public, just exactly what these shows want. This then encourages current clients to examine the sanitation procedures in the salons they patronize, and potential clients have a reason to hesitate when considering becoming a client in a professional salon.

The reality is that salons are safe and clean if routine sanitation and disinfecting practices are followed and that a high degree of sanitation is maintained in the majority of salons. Actually, wise salon owners and professionals can take this negative press and use it to their advantage. These concerns can bring opportunities for internal and external marketing for salons and spas who practice proper sanitation. *Proper sanitation practices can be one of the most effective marketing tools a salon or spa can use.*

INFECTION CONTROL AS A MARKETING TOOL

In a spa concept nail spa, conscientious and consistent infection control practices can be interpreted by the client as professional, up-to-date, and caring. The client will consciously or unconsciously think, "These people know what they are doing, and they really care about me" when she sees prevention procedures. The practicing professional and the salon or spa are seen as prioritizing client safety. Yes, the practice of sanitation and disinfection is marketing and an important contributor to the growth of the business aside from meeting health and state board requirements. Clients can be attracted and maintained by prevention efforts.

Marketing infection control can be a rewarding and inexpensive clientele expansion tool. The method? First, *tell* the clients at every opportunity what and why sanitation practices are being done and why, then consistently perform them within their sight. The opportunities are many! Second, subtly include sanitation practices in advertising and marketing materials. Examples are as follows:

- In the *new client brochure*, place a short paragraph that starts with "Because we care…" explaining that the nail spa is using "clean techniques" to guard their safety.

- Ads in the *newspaper or yellow pages* can contain a short, informative phrase, such as "We use clean techniques for the safety of our clients," or "Sanitation is a priority" in the ad. Those who are concerned will be attracted to it, and others who were previously unaware will recognize it as an indication of the salon or spa's commitment to their safety.

- Use subtle *signage* in the salon to draw attention to the use of procedures to protect clients, such as the placement of a statement, framed and in view of the client, at the scrub sink in the nail spa.

- Use *prevention procedures* in the presence of the clients so they recognize infection control standards are being maintained on their behalf. Spray and cleanse the nail table while the client is preparing to leave. Retrieve implements from a container marked "Sanitary Implements," and place dirty ones in a container marked "Prepare for Sanitation" or clean, and place them in a disinfectant solution in their view.

- Professionals can regularly *explain and discuss* the use of infection control procedures with their clients. A new client can be told, "We require a preservice scrub as a part of our infection control procedures to protect you and our professionals as well as to prepare your nails and skin for the service. Each time you come to visit, you will be scrubbing your hands, prior to sitting down at the table. Let me show you how it is done."

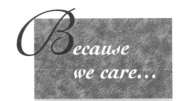

Because we care...

We, the professionals at XX Salon, use clean technique and hospital-grade infection control to safeguard you, our valued clients. If you have any questions, please ask your professional.

Thank you
The Management
XX Salon

My former salon, Nailtique, in Strongsville, Ohio, is an example of the contribution sanitation marketing can make toward your salon's success. I opened the salon, with my daughter, a veteran nail tech. We incorporated the preservice client scrub into the entrance routine and used obvious infection control practices throughout our procedures. We discussed the system with our clients and carried through with a firm commitment to the system.

Our commitment to sanitation procedures was mentioned in our client information, right down to a small transparency on the window of the door. (It was provided by the sanitation system we used.) The reactions of the clients were amazingly verbal. They were pleased and discussed their observations of the infection control practices with their friends. Their friends came in as clients and sent their friends. Many told horror stories about their observations in other salons. Their remarks to us and recommendations to their friends showed open respect for our professionalism and a confidence in our skills. This happened as a result of subtle marketing techniques about something that we performed automatically!

As a result of the recommendations of our clients, we were featured in a half-page article in the *Cleveland Plain Dealer* with the focus on our sanitation practices entitled, "Choosing Your Nail Salon," (Cleveland Plain Dealer). The influx of clients after the article was a great boost for a new nail salon; many came because of our obvious commitment to sanitation. Our little four-professional salon grew quickly.

CHOOSING SAFE NAIL SALON AN IMPORTANT TASK TODAY

If your nails are a mess, you may want a professional miracle worker to bring them to perfection.

But new health concerns about HIV, hepatitis B or even a nail fungus may govern how a nail salon is selected. How do you find one you can trust, that utilizes sanitary procedures to ensure that disease is not transmitted from instruments to clients?

Janet McCormick, a consultant to nail salons who also was a dental hygienist for 20 years, suggests that you ask questions before making an appointment.

"Conscientious salons will be happy to tell you about their sanitation procedures," McCormick said. "The professional nail industry is encouraging clients to insist on sanitary conditions in the salons. They would love to get rid of the few 'bad apples' which attract derogatory media attention. Consumer awareness would quickly put them where they belong: out of business."

In Ohio, nail salons are regulated by the State Board of Cosmetology. All nail technicians must be licensed by the board, which means they have been trained in sanitary procedures.

Tom Ross, administrative assistant to the director of the state board of cosmetology, says that all manicure implements must be scrubbed with hot soapy water and then sterilized in a disinfectant before being used on each client. Also, the finger bowl should be immersed for 10 minutes in a disinfecting solution before being used with a new client. Even the electrical wheel that is used on artificial nails must be taken apart and sterilized before re-use with another client.

Any implement that cannot be sterilized such as an emery board should be discarded after use or given to the client.

McCormick suggests first checking among your friends who use a professional manicurist on the conditions in the salons they use. Some questions to ask:

• Do you have to wash your hands prior to the service?

Technicians and clients are both required to wash their hands, preferably with an antimicrobial soap prior to the service.

The salon's answer to this question is an indication of its policies on sanitation, McCormick said. If a salon does not require the client to wash her hands, it likely is not taking sanitation seriously.

• Does the technician use clean instruments and emeries on each client?

Salons are required to sanitize all implements before they are used on the next client. McCormick says nail stations should have an implement sanitizer in close proximity to the technician. She suggests that a hospital grade disinfectant be used. There should also be separate storage for the sanitized and dirty implements.

• Is the salon clean?

The overall cleanliness of the salon indicates the attitude of the technicians to sanitation. Usually a messy and dirty salon will indicate poor or non-existent sanitation procedures. McCormick said.

You want a "yes" to all of these questions, McCormick says, or don't consider patronizing the salon.

McCormick recommends then calling the salon directly and asking:

• Tell me about your sanitation procedures.

Responses to this question should include disinfecting implements and table surfaces between clients and requiring the client and technician to wash their hands prior to the service. "If these steps are not included, mark the salon off the list," she said.

- What are your policies on the use of emeries?

A sanitary salon will give one of several acceptable answers:
1) New emeries are used, then thrown away or given to the client;
2) Sanitizable emeries are used only once then disinfected;
3) A custom kit of emeries is provided for each client.

Even with the new health concerns raised about some nail salons, a spokesman for the Centers for Disease Control in Atlanta says no cases of AIDS have been reported where the virus was contracted from a nail salon.

AREAS OF DISEASE CONTROL IN A SALON

Prevention of disease within a salon or spa should be a comprehensive process, the collective practices for protecting the client and professionals from the transfer of disease. Five areas of focus exist, each with a somewhat different approach to their prevention activities, but all focus on their particular aspect of disease control. Following are the areas:

- *Environmental sanitation* — The general cleanliness and neatness of the surroundings in a salon or spa
- *Preservice scrub* — A basic requirement for the client and professional to scrub her hands before sitting at the manicure station
- *In-service disinfection practices* — Disinfection procedures within the skill routine
- *Surface disinfection* — A disinfection routine for the top of the nail station table
- *Implement disinfection* — An immersion disinfection routine for reusable implements

The basic purpose for disease control in a nail spa is simple — the prevention of the transfer of disease. A spa professional believes in, understands, and is dedicated to carrying through this process for the protection of the client and herself and for the protection of the reputation of the place she works. In doing so, she is also marketing her nail spa.

Environmental Sanitation

Clients consider environmental sanitation to be a strong indicator of the salon's sanitation procedures. Messiness and dust bother many clients and can initiate a feeling of uneasiness. Conversely, clients like the feeling of security that clean, neat, and orderly surrounding give them and will say so in exit surveys and to their friends. For these reasons, nail spas must seriously look at the condition of their working environment as "internal marketing" procedures, and as everyone's responsibility. Successful nail spas are *clean nail spas*.

The products used for cleaning in any personal service business are important contributors to environmental cleanliness, but especially in businesses where the person is touched. All of these products must contain disinfection ingredients. For instance, surface cleaners must have disinfection qualities and not just mechanically clean the surface. Even the floor cleaners need to have disinfection properties. The labels will state their capabilities, and it is the purchaser's responsibility to find these products for the nail spa. At the same time, the purchaser must be stringently aware of their gentleness on and appropriateness for the surfaces they clean. Luckily, these products are readily available now, even in the grocery stores, though the more effective ones are purchased through the janitorial supplier. They are also less expensive than those in the grocery stores because they are in concentrated form. They no longer leave a hospital-type disinfectant odor, but do leave a clean presence and odor.

"Awareness" and "action" combined are the key. If we are always aware of wayward messiness and acting quickly to straighten it and establish good basic cleaning procedures, our salons will always convey a feeling of safety and caring attentiveness to our clients.

Preservice Scrub

The client scrub is a health issue. Most state regulatory agencies have a statement in their sanitation standards that requires the professionals and clients to "wash their hands" prior to a manicure service. The details of this requirement varies from state to state, but highly professional salons and spas will incorporate it into their sanitation practices as a matter of routine sanitary procedure.

Many contagious diseases are contracted through contact—colds, influenza, fungus, scabies, to name a few—according to the Centers for Disease Control and Prevention in Atlanta, Georgia. As professionals, we should consider the preservice scrub very basic to our protection from the transfer of disease. The client scrub may be considered a bottom line issue: a salon that routinely uses a preservice scrub will have fewer sick days and fewer miserable days for the professionals, and, of course, everyone benefits financially.

The client scrub is a marketing issue, also. A client who is already aware of proper sanitation basics will notice when these practices are lacking, and will consciously or subconsciously be concerned about other disease control practices in the salon. She may search out another salon with better disinfection practices. Conversely, the presence of the preservice scrubbing routine can be seen by her as an indication of good prevention procedures and instill in her a confidence toward other practices in the salon. Even the less knowledgeable clients are more aware of overall disease control practices now and are more attuned to the basics in personal services, such as washing their hands.

Scrubbing is not only for clients. State regulations usually require that professionals cleanse their hands before a service to prevent contaminating a new client's hands with the microorganisms from the last client or from between-service activities. Cleansing also prevents the professionals from being exposed to microbes.

Many clients have patronized other salons that did not practice these procedures. Therefore, professionals must train them to scrub at their first visit. Of course, an effective sanitation procedure is not just a quick hand wash. It has specific steps and the clients must be trained to do them. A clean nail brush is used in the steps, then cleansed, disinfected, and stored in a marked, clean container awaiting the next use. Further, the hand cleanser used in our nail spas should say "antimicrobial" on the label, indicating a broader spectrum of protection than the "antibacterial" products.

The alcohol-based products are not as broad spectrum in protection as other just-as-safe-for-use products that are available to us as working professionals. Further, if a manicurist uses them all day as her cleansing product, the product will cause her hands to dry. I would look for another convenient product, even better, have a sink in the room, if possible, to allow handwashing with a professional lotion-based antimicrobial hand soap.

If a spa professional prefers to use hand cleansers at the table between clients, there are certain considerations:

> She must brush wash her hands several times a day with an antimicrobial soap.
> She must use a paper towel after cleansing with a waterless hand cleanser to remove the debris.
> She must cleanse in the sight of the client to maintain credibility.

Demonstrating the Preservice Scrub. It is important that you personally train your client in the correct method and not just "send" her to the wash stand. Otherwise she will cleanse her hands incompletely at later visits. (Fig. 13–1)

After the client has completed her information, escort her to the wash station to train her in a preservice hand scrub method. (Use this term as it is more "official" than the label of "washing" her hands.)

Say to her, "Please come with me so I can show you our preservice hand scrubbing method. When you do this, it will cleanse your hands *as well as prepare them for the products we will be using during the service.*" The latter phrase should cancel any feelings she may have that her hands are 'sufficiently clean, thank you!'

Turn on the water and adjust the temperature. The temperature of the water heater is primary to this.

At the wash station: Demonstrate on yourself the use of the brush, the drying method, and the exit from the room.

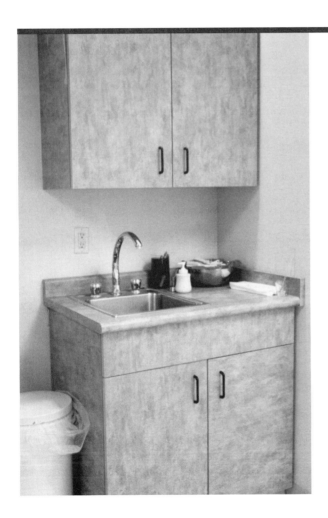

Figure 13-1

A preservice hand scrub area.

1. Wet your hands, and apply an antimicrobial soap and work the lather into the hands. (Fig. 13–2)

2. Wet a *clean* nail brush and place antimicrobial soap on it. Brush under the free edges of your nails and along the cuticles of every finger. (Figs. 13–3 and 13–4)

3. Rinse the brush and place it in the container clearly marked "Used Brushes," then thoroughly rinse your hands.

4. Dry your hands according to the method the salon uses, then demonstrate opening the door with the paper towel and dropping it into the disposal unit. (Fig. 13–5)

Hand the client a clean brush and watch her cleanse her hands. Mention clearly that she should spend at least 10 seconds lathering her hands before going to the brush step, paying close attention to the free edges and cuticles. Handwashing is effective because the friction of rubbing your hands together loosens microbes from your skin and traps them in the lather. Then, when the lather is rinsed down the drain, the microbes go along with it.

Comfortably hot or warm water is preferable because it is more pleasant and more readily removes the lotion soap after the washing proce-

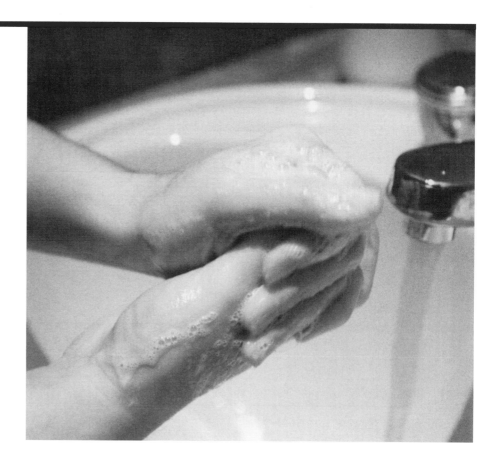

Figure 13-2

Hands are washed with an antimicrobial soap.

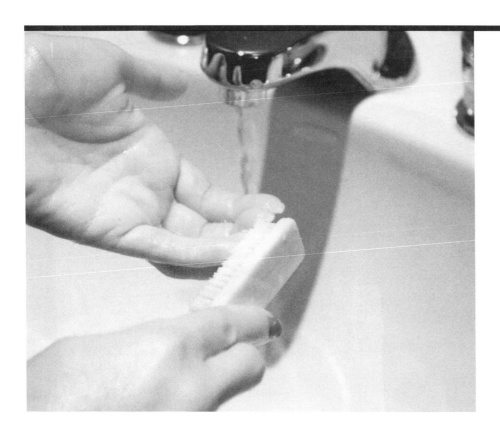

Figure 13-3

Use a wet, clean nailbrush under the free edges of the nails

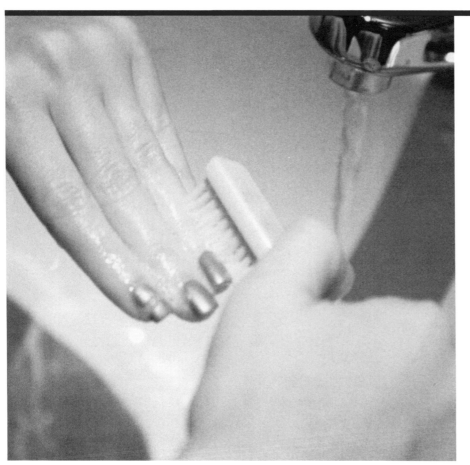

Figure 13-4

Use a nailbrush along the cuticles of every finger.

Figure 13-5

A paper towel is used to open the door and then discarded.

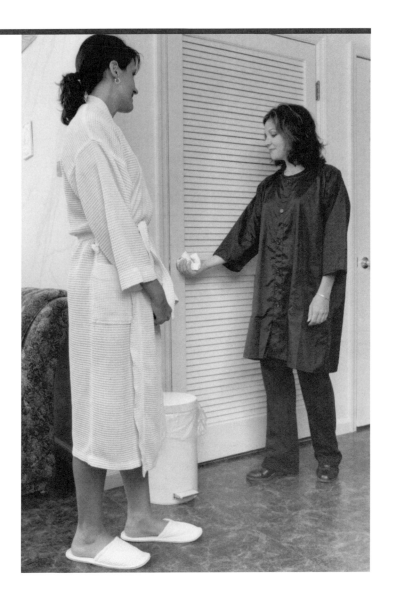

dure. (Water at a wash sink cannot kill microbes because it cannot be warm enough to do so without harming the skin.)

The repeat client is provided a clean brush and sent to the sink to wash. If the spa professional does not cleanse her hands in the direct view of the client, she must use a cleansing method at the table when the client returns. If not, she may feel the spa manicurist is not meeting the same criteria as being requested of her and may resent the procedure. Instead, it should be portrayed as a fully integrated policy, with the spa manicurist cleansing, as the client watches.

Basic In-Service Infection Control Procedures

The central focus of a comprehensive sanitary and disinfection technique is disinfection *at the table and service level*. The salon can be neat and clean, the service areas and surfaces perfect, and everyone's hands clean, but if the client does not see safe table technique used, all other efforts are lost.

Sanitation at the table is a routine. It is a set of procedures placed inside our skill procedures that become a part of them, that should be habitual and necessary for the completion of any service. The procedures are as follows:

- *Entrance*—The client scrubs her hands and comes to the table. The professional cleanses her hands and places clean toweling on the table top. Clean implements are retrieved and placed on the clean table towel. The procedure begins. (Fig. 13–6)
- *During the procedure*—Cleansed and disinfected implements are placed and replaced on the clean towel during the procedure, then placed in a "dirty implement" container at the end of the service for later cleansing and disinfection. The alternative is the immediate brush cleansing, rinse and pat dry, then placement in a disinfection solution. This is in view of the client, if possible, to take advantage of the marketing aspect of sanitation. The occasionally used soak bowl is glass to enable its proper disinfection after use because the plastic manicure soak trays commonly available usually cannot be properly disinfected. Jars and containers are kept clean and dust free and the table surface free of clutter. Disposable supplies are also retrieved from a clean container, then placed/replaced on the table toweling during the procedure.

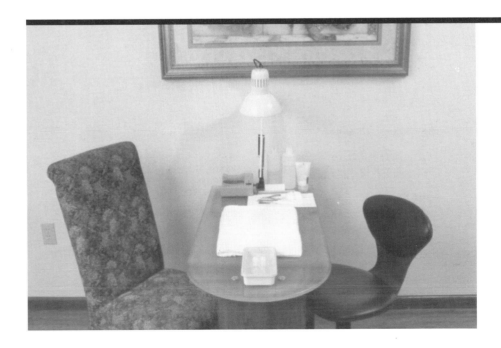

Figure 13-6

The professional places clean towels on the tabletop.

Client antisepsis is maintained, such as cleansing the nail plate prior to application of an enhancement.

- *After the procedure* — Supply containers are wiped clean and replaced in the appropriate storage area. Dirty implements are placed in a "dirty implement" container, or are brush cleansed with soap, pat dried, and placed in an appropriate hospital-grade disinfectant for the length of time suggested in the instructions. Disposable implements and sundries are disposed of immediately or given to the client, if appropriate. Cleanable items, such as towels, are placed in the appropriate closed container or washed in a hot water wash. The table surface is disinfected and "closed" according to the salon policy. (Fig. 13–7) Implements are retrieved from the disinfectant with tongs, rinsed, dried, and placed in a "clean implement" container.

"Closed." A nail spa can ruin its whole image of neatness, cleanliness, and sanitation, basic requirements for marketing sanitation procedures, by the way the stations are left between clients. When a client

Figure 13-7

Implements and the table are properly disinfected after use.

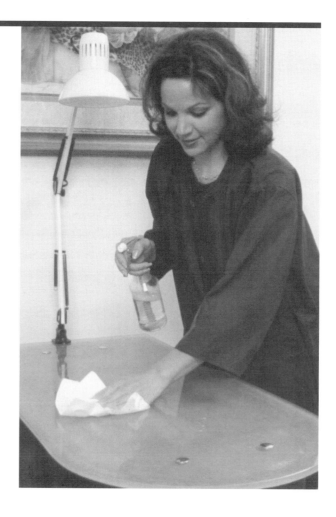

is escorted to the table where she will be sitting, she wants to find a table and chair waiting for *her*, with a neat and clean welcome, not a disarrayed table with obvious remnants of the past client. For that reason, the post service routine should be a quick, easy, and thorough readiness for the next client.

This routine begins with how the professional works during her services. A messy professional will say, "I don't have time for 'closing' my station," and she doesn't—because she works messy, spreading her work space with bottles, implements and papers. She'll say, "I don't have the room to put all this away." This is usually *not* true, she is just unorganized, but if it is, something needs to be modified in her work area. A neat and clean station between clients is an important image issue and must be accomplished.

Usually, however, the issue is the work habits of the professional, and must be dealt with at the very basis of her routines. One suggestion is working in "units," the collection of the products and supplies for each section of a skill together so they can be retrieved and replaced in one movement. For instance, if the professional is at the building step of her enhancement, the product requirements for this step should be all together, possibly on a nice porcelain flat dish that can be found at the emporiums. The powder is in a closed 1-ounce container, which is clean and neat looking. The liquid dappen dish is there, along with a dispenser of liquid that is only large enough to hold one day's liquid. Her application brush is there, in a dust-free holder, plus any other products that the professional uses during her building procedure.

This unit of products can be retrieved in one movement, provided the professional has prepared it at the beginning of the day, and replaced in one movement at the end of the building section of the procedure; then the finishing unit is retrieved and replaced for its section of the procedure. The prep step products and equipment are also together as a work unit. Working in units is clean and neat, even attractive to the client. The table is easy to clear at the end of the service and can be left in a standard 'between clients' appearance, termed 'closed' here for our purposes.

Closed is a standard appearance that has been defined for the station for whenever the professional is absent from the station and for between clients for the new client to see as she is seated. The appearance is defined by the manager or by the unanimous definition by the professionals. Whatever it is, it is the only accepted appearance of the station whenever a service is ended and between clients. No set standard is defined other than what the nail spa decides will fit its image and storage capabilities.

The table top may be the following: A ceramic lotion dispenser, a ceramic polish remover dispenser, a decorative glass container (with a top on it) for cotton or 2″ x 2″ squares for polish removal and other purposes, a card holder, and a folded towel lying in the service area, possibly with a folder paper service towel on it or under it. (Fig. 13–8) The table top is cleanable and unstained, and the towels are top quality, unstained and in good condition. When a client approaches the table she will see it as neat and obviously clean.

The secret to the successful use of work units and a closed routine is education. The starting professional is trained in working this way and it easily becomes routine for her. The working professional who already has a work routine, possibly a less organized one, will be more of a challenge. The dedicated professional will work into the routine, successfully; good luck with the resistant one.

Surface Disinfection

Surface disinfection involves all the surfaces in the salon, but the most important and a step up in procedures is the surface of the work stations. (All others can be maintained with good environmental disinfection procedures.) *Every station should be sprayed and cleaned after every client*

Figure 13-8

The area is clean with unstained, top quality towels ready for the client.

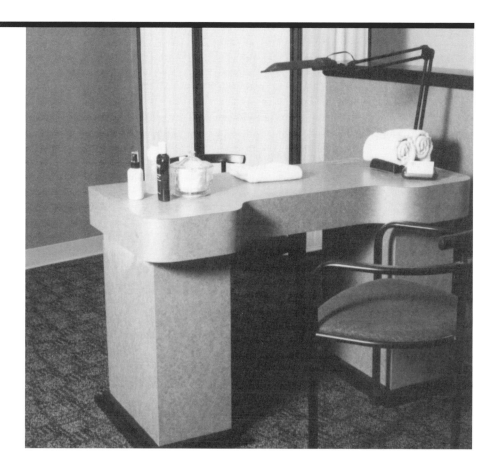

with a good surface disinfectant that is designed for our industry. (Windex is not a product for use on our tables.)

Dust is inherent to our work, as is protein debris such as cuticles and nail filings. These particles can transfer and breed disease. Further, clients are offended by the lack of responsibility a salon demonstrates when this debris is not removed.

Basic housekeeping is important to prevent this happening along with in-service procedures such as using work units and a good close procedure. The clear table top will allow easy and effective cleaning, allowing the client to feel like the area is ready and especially clean, just for her. A nail spa integrates procedures, such as work units and designing an acceptable close that will support feelings such as these for each and every client.

Implement Disinfection

Explanation of the basic procedures for disinfecting implements can bear some repetition to prevent any misunderstanding of the procedure and to reinforce a good habit. Standard procedures are as follows:

- *Implements must be cleansed before placing them in the disinfectant* — Many conscientious nail professionals use their implements, then drop them immediately into a disinfection unit that is kept on the table. The problem? They have misunderstood the role of debris in infection control. The debris left on implements will eventually overburden the disinfectant, rendering it useless for the purposes of disinfection. The result? The professional has a false sense of safety and the implements are not disinfected. The disinfectant is not doing its job. Actually, under these conditions, the disinfectants can ultimately *breed* microbes, if the it is not changed in time. Proper procedure is to cleanse the implement, rinse it off, pat dry, and place it in the disinfectant.
- *The implements must be **brushed clean*** — Soaping and rinsing an implement can leave minute amounts of debris on an implement. Protein debris, such as nail clippings or minute pieces of cuticle, become hardened by disinfectants and become a type of shield for microbes against the action of the disinfectant. The easiest and most certain method for complete removal of this debris is vigorous cleansing of the implements with a *nail brush* during their cleansing with soap and water.

- *The implements must be rinsed before placing them in the disinfectant*—The soaps and detergents used during the precleansing step can cancel the disinfection properties of many disinfectants. Debris from the soaps or detergents must be rinsed off the implements before they are placed in the disinfectant solution.

- *Wet implements can dilute the disinfectant*—The nail professional must pat dry her implements after cleansing and rinsing them, before placing them in the disinfectant. Otherwise, there may be a change in the disinfectant beyond adequate strength. The pat-dry movement is a quick motion and is it worth the small effort to ensure prevention of dilution.

- *Implements must be rinsed when removed from the disinfectant*—When the nail professional habitually removes her implements from the disinfectant with her hands or immediately begins to use them without rinsing them, she is subjecting herself to overexposure to the disinfection chemicals. These products are "pesticides-for-tiny-pests," and subjecting ourselves to chronic exposure to even the most mild disinfectant is unwise.

- *Proper dilution of the disinfectant with water is important to effective disinfection*—The products must be mixed as the label directs or the disinfection process will not be successful. This is not the place to economize by diluting the product more than it says in the directions.

- *"Change when cloudy" is not an adequate signal for replenishing disinfection solutions*—Cloudiness in a solution indicates contamination, the solution is no longer capable of disinfection and may be breeding microbes. It is debris and other contaminants in the solution, possibly even microbes. We should not wait for the solution to reach this state, but change it on a regular basis. However, the time for becoming cloudy will be different for all salons and spas.

  To determine when to routinely change a disinfectant in a nail spa, use the product as usual and note when the cloudiness becomes apparent. For example, at 3 days, the solution begins to be cloudy. In this salon, the solution should be routinely changed at 2 days. One professional salon, for instance, may only need to change the disinfectant every 5 to 7 days; however, it must be done before it begins to show cloudiness.

Spa Manicuring for the Salon and Spa

WHAT'S IN IT FOR ME?

Sometimes the most important marketing of sanitation practices needs to be done to the nail professionals. The benefits for using a well-designed disease control routine must be personalized for them or they may not have a long-standing commitment to the practices. Several benefits can be found for each individual professional using good asepsis techniques.

1. The individual professional will lose fewer work days. Days lost to illness can dramatically affect a professional's lifestyle.

2. The professionals can feel safer in working on the general public. How many times have we wondered about working on a particular client, but could not avoid it?

3. The professional will achieve a new level of respect. Clients voice their new respect for a professional who uses obvious techniques to protect them.

4. The clients will recommend the nail spa professional to their friends. When sweeps month and its nasty nail salon segment airs next year, this professional's clients will *brag* to their friends and send them into the nail spa for safe services.

5. The professional will be positively differentiated from others. This professional is different from those down the street who work like those on TV, and the clients can see it.

6. The professional's take-home pay will increase due to the added clients. More clients mean more money in the pockets of busy professionals.

7. Good-bye, Greenies! That problem will not exist at this professional's table.

8. The professional can welcome state board visits with a smile and sincere greeting. Why worry? This professional knows she is within the regulations.

Committed nail spa professionals will see these benefits come to them individually and, in turn, to the nail spa.

NO TIME FOR SANITATION

Sadly, sanitation is an area in which some professionals rebel and make "I don't have time for all this!" statements. A workable system can be tailored to the needs of the individual professionals, as well as to those of large nail spas. However, a very busy professional may need two or more sets of reusable implements to allow proper cleansing/disinfection rotations.

The system designer is responsible for designing a system as convenient and simple as possible, though effective, then providing implementation through training. This training should be designed to establish good sanitation habits within the professionals' routines.

Proper sanitation is a series of *habits*, that's all—habits that we can ingrain into our routine easily and effectively. If we are committed to the procedures, we will place them in our routines, do them, and be glad we did. Soon they become second nature and valuable to execution of the table routine...and an excellent marketing tool for a spa concept salon.

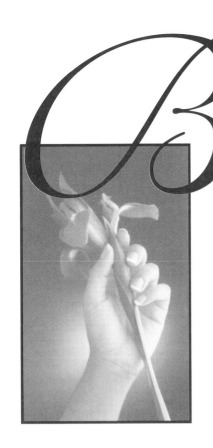

Building Your Clientele and Income

14

OBJECTIVES

At the end of this chapter, you should be able to:

- Reappoint clients at the end of an appointment.
- Build a loyal and eager clientele.
- Sell a high percentage of home care products against the gross.
- Improve the client's hand and nails through home care.

The spa professional who has reached the pinnacle of success in her career has accomplished several things: she has reached a high percentage of bookings with a high number of them as regular clients, and her retail (home care) percentage is 20% or more. Careful attention to the "success points" during each client's visit can make this happen.

Success points are locations within the procedures when suggestions are made and affirmations are noted concerning future appointments and retail purchases. A professional who educates herself on these points, then integrates them in a natural and nurturing manner into her clients' care will have a large clientele and sell a high number of home care products.

It is understandable that so many manicurists shun the thought of retailing and hesitate to ask for the next appointment (though not excusable). After all, we consider ourselves artists, not salespeople, and might even regard selling as embarrassing or demeaning. "Let the receptionist do it," we say. The client will *ask* for another appointment, if she really wants one. "I feel pushy when I come right out and ask her to reappoint," we say. We give her every avenue of escape she needs!

Unfortunately, our reluctance to "sell" home care products and to ask our clients to make their next appointment, or even better, to set up a program or purchase a package of services, hinders our clientele growth—and the resulting income—to much less than what is its potential. To overcome this we must feel comfortable about "selling" and asking a client to return.

SELLING IS A CLIENT SERVICE

When a client purchases services from a nail spa, she is anticipating:
- Superlative services
- Immediate improvement
- Effects of the services to last longer than those from another salon

These expectations can be met only if the service skills are superlative and appropriate products are sent home with her to extend the effects of the service and to continue the improvements. If the effects are only short term—most last a very short time if good home care products are not sent home with her—the client will become discouraged and return only a few times, if at all. With quality home care products that support her needs, the effects will be extended, improvements in the conditions of the nails and skin will be evident, and the client will return regularly to a professional who has provided a great service for her.

WHY IS REAPPOINTING IMPORTANT?

We have all seen her—the technician who just never develops a good clientele. She is discouraged, poor and usually quickly out of the business. We have also seen the one whose clientele grew from zero to capacity in 3 to 4 months. Assuming that these professionals are in a salon with the same growth opportunities in training, promotion, and traffic, what is the difference between them? If personality is the key as some will say, what about the technician who has the personality of a barracuda and clientele on a wait list? One key is getting the client back in, and she does it. She accomplishes a commitment to reappoint early in the appointment, or makes certain it is done when the client goes to the desk.

No professional or salon can depend on a constant flow of new clients to fill the appointment book except possibly in a few day spas where packages fill the chairs every day. But new clients cannot keep the doors to a salon open. Regulars are the mainstay for paying the bills in this business, even the day spas. It costs two to three times more to attract a new client than to retain an old one. The established client will also spend twice as much on services and home care at an appointment than a new one will, if she is approached correctly.

That Dreaded Selling

I developed my methods for reappointing and retailing while working as a dental hygienist, telling the client "what-why-when-how and how much." It did not come naturally to me. I had to learn through trial and error.

I started selling at the dental chair when I was a dental hygienist, on a whim. (Selling in dentistry is called 'case presentation' and is traditionally done by the dentist.) My dentist boss was uncomfortable reciting prices and educating patients on their need for high ticket procedures and, as a result, the practice was suffering financially. One day, I decided to try doing a case presentation. Why not? I could not do any worse than he did. I explained to a patient why the crowns and bridges were needed, then made an appointment. The first sale was easy, so I tried it on a couple of clients. It worked reasonably well. My boss was pleased, so, before he got used to me doing it for no extra compensation, I made a proposal to him. He gladly gave up the chore in exchange for paying me a small percentage. After all, he was not doing well with it. Why not let me try? I was excited! Many of those cases were over $10,000!

After I took over the chore, I decided to use the formal method of presentation as they train the dentists in dental school. I sat down with the patients and went over their needs in detail. It was time consuming and difficult because I was heavily booked at the chair. I was so stressed that several times I developed hives! I could not get the words out, and when I did I was uncomfortable and sounded unsure of my facts. I was discouraged and my boss was disappointed. It was not as easy as it had been the first day. Was that a fluke?

Then I discussed the challenge with my husband, a sales manager, who explained how easy it could be. "The most successful selling is *inside* a service, as you did that first day," he said. "You've got it made. As long as you believe in what you're selling and are meeting the patient's needs, he or she won't feel a "hard sell" and will recognize a need for the product. Use your treatment plans during the time you have them in your room with you as you did before," he said. "It's more natural that way."

He was right. Before long, I had more than doubled my income, the practice was doing very well, my boss bought a new house, and the patients had healthier teeth. I was on a roll!

When I left dentistry, however, I failed to take my "sales" skills with me. I did not recognize the connection with the clients' well-being that I had seen in dentistry. I fell into the same rut that other nail technicians were in…retailing embarrassed me. My percentage was the same as most every technician's, around 5% to 7%, and often even less unless I was really interested in some product we were selling. It took years for me to awaken to the similarity between the two situations.

When I did, however, it was with a jolt. It occurred to me one day while driving to the salon. (Sadly, it was *years* after I became a technician.) I realized I could give myself an income increase using those old techniques I had developed long ago. I refined my retail menu around my service menu and entered a new era. There were many days my retail actually matched my services! The least I did was 25%. The obvious improvements in my client's hands and nails were seen by their friends and my clientele grew quickly as a direct result. Let me explain how it works:

POINTS: THIS IS HOW IT WORKS

Point One: Client Analysis

This is the treatment plan part of my former job and the 'identify the client's needs" part of selling techniques. Analysis is the most important step in the reappointment and retailing procedures. During the analysis, you examine and discuss the condition of the client's skin and nails, then *educate her* on how you can help. You tell her what you see, and how you and she can deal with it. Home care is described, future appointments are suggested, and the end results defined.

Spa professionals who omit this step usually sell only 5% to 7% of their gross in retail, and as few as only 50% of the new clients reappoint, depending on the technical skills of the manicurist. Not only do manicurists miss out on the additional income because they sell only what clients request, even the reappointing clients may disappear from the appointment book. They become discouraged over the condition of their nails (no improvement) and the lack of lasting effects of the service between appointments.

Let's use an example, the client with dry cuticles. During the analysis, the spa manicurist draws attention to her dry cuticles and suggests a goal that can be achieved. For instance, "You and I can take care of this. You work on them at home, and I'll work on them here. They'll be exactly what you want them to be if we work together! We'll start today with a hydrating manicure, and I'll show you what to do at home. You will love your hands in a few weeks!"

During the same discussion, you project to her the results that she will see after this appointment, "You won't have these rough edges after today as I'll clean up the dry areas and soften the rest," and the next, "You'll see improvement this week with the cuticle treatment. Next week I will do another hydration, plus some exfoliation to bring up the new cuticle underneath." Mention the goal—healthy, smooth cuticles—and that you will help her achieve it. Look her in the eye, touch her hands and say, "*We* can do this!"

Proceed then to home care—her part in achieving the goal. Describe the benefits of a suggested product, show her how to use it, and *bring it to the table*. You might say, "We have a product that will improve this moisture in your cuticles dramatically when you use it regularly at home. It's an aromatherapy oil with tiny molecules that absorb easily and provide excellent moisturization. Let me show you how to use it, and I'll get you one to take home." Then, get up and get it. (Fig. 14–1) Other products, such as an appropriate lotion, should be included in the process.

You also prepare the client to purchase other needed products. You say, "Next week we'll get you started on a home care cuticle exfoliation treatment. With the use of the oil and that product at home you'll really see these manicures making a difference quickly!"

You will need to know everything possible about the products to recommend them: how they work, what ingredients they contain, the results to be expected, and how often they must be used for optimum results (see Chapter 11).

Point Two: Instruct and Demonstrate

To demonstrate your belief in a product's efficacy, it is critical that you use it on the client during the service. Coach the client on how to properly use the product. For instance, if the client has dry, cracked cuti-

Figure 14-1

Suggest products for home care use to the client.

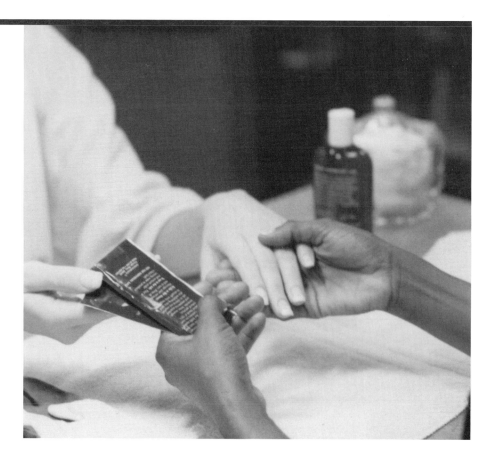

Spa Manicuring for the Salon and Spa

cles, use an alpha hydroxy acid cuticle cream or aromatherapy oil during the treatment, according to what is seen during the analysis, and brief her on the product's benefits and proper application procedure. (Fig. 14–2) For the aromatherapy cuticle oil, you might say, "You'll need to use this product morning and evening to nourish and hydrate your cuticles for best results. I suggest you apply it like this. Of course, you can use it more often if you wish." For the alpha hydroxy acid product, you would explain how it promotes softening and exfoliation.

Point Three: Verify

Raise the client's awareness of her needs and your ability to meet them by mentioning future appointments and the home care products throughout the service when possible and natural. For instance, "Your dry hands are in much better shape now *since the sloughing and hydration treatments*. Isn't this great! They'll be even better *when you use the lotion I suggested at home*. We'll do another hydration next week after you've worked on them at home and you'll begin to see new hands!" Notice I used the words "since" and "when," not "if."

There is no single appropriate time or method during a procedure to verify a client's needs; verify them at every opportunity, in a natural way that fits into her service.

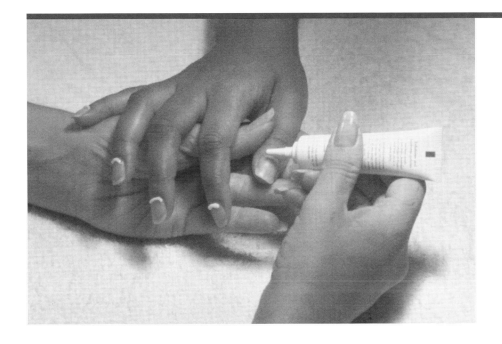

Figure 14-2

Show the client how to properly use each product you suggest.

PRODUCT PRICE POINTS

Some clients will have questions about the prices of the products. If the professional knows her client well, she will probably have a good idea when or if to mention this: a new client will somehow let her know if it is important. However, professionals should not get bogged down in cost issues.

Remember that these clients are already purchasing discretionary services by seeking services in the nail spa and are also declaring their desire for nice hands and nails by being there. I call this the "open purse theory." I suggest that a nail spa professional visualize each spa manicuring client as sitting there holding her purse open and saying: "I want you to give me new hands. I have said this by coming through the door and sitting down at your station. *Now*. Reach in and take the money needed to accomplish this." If a spa professional visualizes her spa manicure clients in this way, she will lose her fear of selling.

A professional who is uncomfortable about stating prices can mention how long the product will last: "This should last you about 3 months," before stating the price. Most products are designed to last that long if used according to directions. This discomfort is usually unjustified, however. If the produce menu is carefully chosen to fit the niche of the nail spa, the prices should not be a problem for these clients. After all, they have already made the statement that they want nice hands by coming into the salon.

Another important factor is *learning when to be appropriately silent*. Many professionals talk too much during a service, believing that is what their clients want. They might talk about everything *except* the client's hands, nails, skin, and feet. Sometimes, the subjects are even inappropriate. Instead, try this successful service scenario: stop, look, and listen, then recommend. Clients come to a nail spa to improve their appearance and relax. The professional should *look at their hands* and ask questions about them, not about their divorce or their kids. Listen to what they have to say about their nails and hands. Then, tell them what you observe, what they need today and at home, how to use the recommended products, when and for what services they need to reappoint, and what results they can expect.

Relaxation techniques will enable them to think about their hands and skin, not about their problems and stresses. For example, "I'm going to do a great massage on your hands now, so I want you to close your eyes and take three deep breaths, holding each for 2 seconds, then let them out slowly—the massage works better and you'll enjoy it more. Now…"

In this scenario, the client's service results will be better, she will listen and think about what has been said, and she will be more apt to purchase the products she needs to continue her treatments at home. All this should be performed with a friendly demeanor and attitude.

Point Four: Closing the Sale

After identifying the client's needs and suggesting and demonstrating the home care, you will *psychologically* transfer the products to her ownership. This is done during the analysis step, then reinforced with the "whens" throughout the service. It is a psychological transfer of product, not yet a transfer of money. The product is placed next to the client on her side of the table after the benefits have been discussed. When you are using it on her, point to it and remind her that "this is what I am using, and here is how you will use it." As she moves from questions about the benefits to questions about how she uses it, say, "I will put this in a bag for you." Then, do so, immediately if the nail spa is set up for that. (Fig. 14–3)

Many clients will indicate by their movements whether they are ready to purchase a product. Watch for movements like leaning slightly toward the product, or putting her arm next to it, or even reading the

Figure 14-3

Close the sale by answering all questions about benefits and how to use it, then place them in a bag.

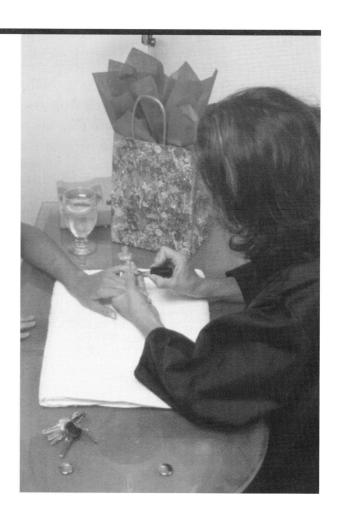

label or smelling the aroma—these are territorial or acceptance movements. If she moves slightly away from it or never looks at it, that means she is not ready yet to decide to purchase. Still place it next to her during her time at the table. Reinforce the benefits whenever it is being used during the service. At the close of the appointment, suggest it be included in her total for the day. She may be ready to purchase it then.

Another reason technicians often do not sell is the small amount their commission appears to be. Many mistakenly see 10% to 20% of their retail gross as minuscule and too small for the effort required. This is true if their retail sales are 5% to 7%. (The professionals sold so little in my early salons that I paid it quarterly.) However, I challenge you to try these methods. Even 10% of $100 per day in retail, an easily achievable goal with the right products, will add up significantly each pay day—not to mention having happier clientele and more of them returning; $10 per day will soon become a significant amount!

Reappointment Language

Reappointment points are interspersed throughout the appointment. During the analysis the professional mentions her future needs and what can be done to achieve her goal. During the service she mentions the results the client will get with this appointment, and what will be done when she returns...again, "when" not "if." Other mentions are how far her nails will grow each week "between appointments," improvements she will see with each service, and when she can expect to see her goal reached, after the suggested services. Any mention of future services that will fit *naturally* into the conversation should be done.

During the appointment, the client will see the improvements and how much she enjoys the service, and will provide "signals" toward reappointing. It is the manicurist's responsibility to verify these signals with affirming comments, as above and if appropriate. The manicurist will sense early in the appointment whether the client will return. Prior to polishing, affirm the next appointment, such as, "Next time you come in I will be doing an (X) treatment and (X) manicure, and you will begin seeing even more dramatic improvements. It will take (amount of time) for the service; when should we set that up?"

It is important for at least one verification of reappointment to be made by the spa professional early in each appointment. During each analysis, the spa manicurist must encourage her client on the progress of her hands toward her goal. "Your nails/hands are really improving! Aren't we doing great? We're a great team!" Then, go right into what will be done at that appointment and the next one. Of course, there are those clients who will not do their part, and this has to be acknowledged and dealt with. After she has learned the analysis skill well, the manicurist will know when a client has not performed her home care. She should be asked if she has missed some applications or has been exposing her hands to an extra amount of environmental negatives.

Reappointing points can take a clientele from small to a nice clientele in 3 months, even if a spa manicurist starts at zero. (This is assuming that clients are coming through the door, of course.) All but a small number of clients will become regulars if the professional is fully trained and she uses the success points. The clients will send their friends, who will send her their friends, who...

All clients should be given the opportunity to become a regular client and to purchase home care products to do their part in the evolution of their hands. Clients using package deals are included in this; even those who have come in on a 1-day visit are potential regulars and should be offered the care and opportunity to become one...unless they live too far away. (But how far is "far?")

A check on home care

One spa manicurist I know requires her neglectful clients to bring in their home care products so she can see that they are using them. They usually change their habits because they do not want to hear her chastisements! She marks their bottles! All this is done in a friendly, caring manner, of course. Encouragement to improve should follow the comments on missing applications of home care.

Availability of Products

We have all run out of products at one time or another. However, no spa manicurist can meet her potential in home care if the shelves are frequently empty. Further, the professionals will become hesitant to make recommendations and the downward spiral begins: no home care, less client improvement, then fewer reappointments, and on and on.

Low inventory is usually a management problem that should be corrected and closely monitored. (Just-in-time inventory control is not an excuse.) If it is a distributor or manufacturer problem, cross them off the supplier list and find a new one. These products are vital to the salon's and professional's income and the well-being and growth of the clientele! Further, when the shelves are well-stocked, clients will be more likely to browse, ask questions, and purchase on impulse. (Fig. 14–4)

Once a professional starts analyzing her client's needs and practices the above home care steps, she will soon see positive results in her clients' nails and skin. Home care recommendations will come naturally to her, her clients' skin and nails will be in better condition with each appointment and, best of all, she will have given herself a raise! Once she starts building reappointments inside the manicures, her clientele and the nail spa's will grow and so will the income.

Figure 14-4

Keeping the shelves fully stocked will allow clientele to browse and shop on impulse.

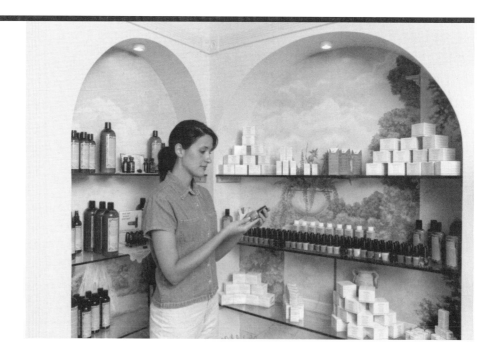

PACKAGING

Nail spas are showing a trend toward *packaging*, one of the appointing traditions of day spas. In a typical spa package, the client spends a block of time experiencing many different services, some of which may be new to her. For this reason, packages are excellent vehicles for building clientele for day spas as they introduce clients to new possibilities for future purchases. Packaged services can be excellent vehicles for building clientele in nail spas also.

There are three types of packaging: the one-time package, the dollar amount package, and the service package. Each is purchased in advance and provides guaranteed clients, cash flow, and marketing opportunities.

One-time packages are purchased usually by significant others, bosses, or children of the client to pamper her and are the most popular package in day spas. They are a group of services, prepackaged or custom choices, typically purchased as a gift for the holidays, a birthday, or anniversary. A typical prepackaged purchase would contain a facial, a spa manicure and pedicure, an herbal wrap, a massage, a shampoo/blow dry hair style, a makeup application, and luxurious lunch. This package is very popular, but there are many to choose from. Package design is only restricted by the imagination of the menu designer.

The *dollar amount packages* are just what they say. The purchaser pays a chosen amount for a gift certificate that has no specified services. The beneficiary can use it as a one time package or spend it over time, just like money, on services of her choice. This package is usually purchased as a gift.

Service packages contain a series of specific services that will be used over time. These are usually purchased by the client who will use them and are the most popular money-maker packages for specialty salons, such as skin care salons. They contain particular services that are repeated and may be offered for a small discount from the regular price, or a "gift with purchase" is provided as an incentive for purchase of the package. A well-known example of service packages is the "10 tans for $X" that are a permanent part of the tanning industry.

Service packages are the mainstay of the skin and body care industries and are an untapped resource for nail spas. When most of us think of packages in our nail salons, we think of the one-time package, such as a manicure/pedicure promotion that is offered as a pampering promotion to introduce pedicures or to increase business during the slow season. Few nail salons offer service packages, though they are tailored perfectly to our clients. An example would be the "six fills for $150" package.

Packages Spell Success

Skin care salons can tell us that service packages can make the difference between mediocre and great success for a salon. Nail salons should note their success with packages. Some of the advantages of packaging services are:

- *Pampering packages are clientele builders*—Clients who are given one-time pampering packages are exposed to the salon; they may never have come in otherwise. This visit can be the first of many appointments, if the client enjoys the services.

- *Dollar amount packages are money in the bank*—Prepayment makes the money available to build on current business, to attract new business, or to hold for future needs. These are wonderful packages to introduce a new client to spa concept manicures and treatments!

- *Dollar amount package clients spend more per service*—When someone else purchases a dollar amount package for her, a client sees the opportunity to spend more. She can purchase retail products with this money also, so many clients really spend money on products.

- *Service packages build loyalty*—Repeat service packages will establish a consumer habit both with the salon and the professionals and will develop an "ownership" of the salon, that is, "my nail salon," or "my technician." This builds loyalty when the services go well. When the package is completed, this client is usually *yours*.

- *A client base is ensured*—These clients patronizing the salon can be counted on for future appointments and retail purchases. Many become repeat package purchasers. Their names and addresses are available for future marketing.

- *The nail spa has the money*—Package money is up-front. The money for the services that may be done over 6 months is in the bank. Invested wisely in the business, this money can bring in more new business. However, careful planning for cash-flow purposes is important.

- *Non-used packages are a bonus to the business*—Many packages are never fully used, making the unused portion available for investment in the future of the salon. However, a wise nail spa professional will seek out a package client who does not use her complete package and perhaps address the reasons it was not used. A happy package purchaser will be a client for a long time to come, and many continue to purchase other packages and services after their first one is finished.

- *Cancellation policies can be easily enforced*—How many times do salons agonize over charging a client for a missed appointment? Or, just take the loss instead of an argument? This is no problem with package clients. A phrase on the accompanying information for the package can have a policy statement that takes care of this problem *ahead of time*. "Missed appointments without a 24 hour notice will be deducted from the package." There is no agonizing here. The policy for the other clients seems more easily reinforced, once this is in place. It is a fairness thing.

Service packages have some unique advantages of their own:

- *A client with a service package can average a higher ticket in retail*— These clients will spend more in retail. They want the full advantage of the repeated services and will be more open to a structured home care program. To fulfill this potential, the professionals must be fully trained in the advantages of home care, product knowledge, analysis procedures, and retailing. Many times these clients will upgrade, actually, if the analysis is done properly.

- *A service package client may tip higher*—Tipping is a controversial issue. If a salon professional accepts tips, the client who has purchased repeat services usually will tip higher than when paying for each visit. The reason may be that the immediate service cost is not as noticeable, or that paying at the end of a service is a habit. The one-time package client may or may not tip at all, and the amount may be high or low.

- *A service package client is in better condition and is easier to service*—This client will be in for her services regularly and will usually perform her home care. Her services consist of less "catch up" and more maintenance and she becomes a participant in her treatment. Her results and therapeutic progress are more predictable. She is more fun to work with!

- *Service package clients appoint in advance*—Clients who prepay are more likely to reappoint as they leave, or become "standings," that is, every Thursday at one. They will build their lives around services that are prepaid.

The restrictions it may place on client analysis is the disadvantage of service packaging. None of us can predict the condition of the client's hands three manicures in advance. However, after a learning curve, most manicurists can foretell a particular client's needs for certain skin and nail conditions enough to design an appropriate package. Still, the best approach may be to educate the client, at the time of purchase, to possible revisions in the package should her skin or nails demand a change in approach.

A well-designed brochure can also deal with this problem, saying that any indication that another service will more appropriately meet her needs will be mentioned to the client. It should also mention that there could be occasions when this will mean an additional fee for a higher cost service.

TREATMENT PROGRAMS

Our best treatment results are shown through "programs," a series of services to which the client commits, achieving and maintaining beautiful skin and nails, from her fingertips to her elbows. These programs are developed through analysis and are as individual as those in the skin care department. The first appointment will show the most dramatic results; the others will follow at a more leisurely pace to complete the trek to the goal. The client will be watching the results closely along the way.

These programs are not the prepaid packages of many esthetics departments. Instead, because clients in nail salons are not accustomed to packaging, *programs* may be the better way to describe them, such as, "Let me tell you about my nail growth program. It's perfect for you and you will have beautiful nails in 6 weeks."

The difference between programs and packages is simple. Programs are not paid in advance as with packages and do not have a set number of visits. In manicuring, it is often best to not sell a series (package) of six prepaid and prenamed manicures or treatments to some clients, placing them within a rigid regimen that would restrict the manicures to those that were previously sold. These may not be appropriate with changes that may occur in the skin and nails between the time the package is sold and the manicures and treatments are performed. Packages restrict the analysis-driven manicure unless the client is prepared to be open to upgrades.

The knowledgeable professional will soon be able to discern which program is best for a particular client who hopes for a specific result. The professional describes the program in detail, involving the client in the trek toward her desired goal. This goal is the greatest advantage of a program—it keeps the client coming in, and the incremental accomplishment toward the goal is her best encouragement for keeping the appointments religiously. The accomplishment of the goal, and its successful maintenance through analysis and the recommended manicures and treatments, is her reward for loyalty for the salon.

Another advantage in describing the treatments as a program is that the client senses a goal and will be more likely to appoint and not miss appointments. Also, she has less of an "I-want-this-right-now" attitude; she will have more patience with the treatments.

Some programs, however, are best sold as prepaid packages, such as the glycolic treatment series. Glycolic treatment produces its most effective results after four weekly treatments, and a package will be more likely to ensure these appointments are faithfully kept.

The spa manicures and hand treatments included in programs will prepare the skin's surface for the needed changes (which you will define), condition the surface, attain the goal, and maintain it once it has been reached. The nail care programs will go hand in hand with the skin care and show equally as impressive results. Home care is a necessity to enhance and maintain our work.

To define and recommend the proper services, you must be familiar with the skin situation you will observe during your analysis, the nail care conditions, and how to deal with them. Your goal is to investigate the possible causes of problems, explain how you can help her with them, involve her in a program that will get her hands and nails in good shape and then show her a dramatic improvement with her first manicure. These recommendations involve decisions on your part as to the program that will provide the very best results for the particular client at the table at that moment. You will then describe them to the client, with the possible results, and proceed from that point.

To develop your client's program, you will, through analysis, include manicures and treatments in a regimen that you will recommend and home care items for the client's partnership in the attainment of the goal. (Those manicures and treatments are discussed in detail in Chapter 5.) These programs must meet four criteria:

1. The client must see dramatic results from the first treatment. She must have immediate hope that she can get the ultimate results she wants.

2. The client must commit to future appointments designed to achieve a targeted result. It is impossible to achieve reliable results with erratically performed services.

3. The program must fit the needs of the individual client. The client with rough, cracked hands will not need the same program as one with chafed, raw hands. The client with weak, frilly nails will not need the same nail care program as the one with hard, brittle nails. For this reason, the effectiveness of the programs depends on your ability to accurately analyze each client's needs.

4. The client must participate in attainment of the goal through a home care regimen.

When you explain a program to a client, make it clear that you will be able to make her hands soft and more attractive in only one manicure and her nails shaped and manicured; however, emphasize that as long as the environmental and lifestyle elements contributing to the problems continue to exist, the condition will return immediately if the program is not maintained. The partnership must continue, your part and hers, in a program designed especially for her hands. You must impress on her that meeting her goal of smooth, soft skin and longer, beautiful nails will require effort from both of you—a true partnership.

TREATMENT PROGRAMS AND PACKAGING = PROFESSIONALISM

Treatment programs and packaging are a true characteristic of "being a spa" in our country and reflect a professionalism far beyond that of current manicure services if they are analysis driven. They can produce dramatic results for most clients with skin and nail problems. Their correct use can bring a whole new meaning to the term "natural nails services" for clients with chronic nail and skin disappointments.

A nail spa with great programs that *work* and skilled professionals that use analysis-driven manicures and treatments and reappointment and home care points will more rapidly develop a clientele of loyal followers, with a high percentage of retention.

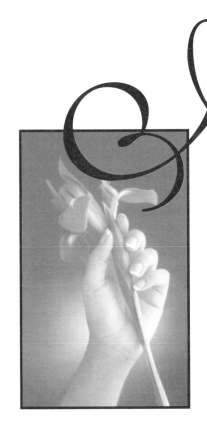

Implementation: Becoming Spa

15

OBJECTIVES

At the end of this chapter, you should be able to:

- Implement spa concept services.
- Design processes for implementing spa manicuring services.

Spa concept is now the standard a salon wants to achieve in its professional care and attitudes, or a professional wishes to implement it at her table. So, does management call a meeting, announce the change, give a class, and try it? Or, does the professional go to the supply house, purchase the products and get on with it? No. Such a simplistic approach will ensure frustration for the management team or the professional and probably failure of the concept. The employees will be sitting with their palms up, saying, "What's the big deal about this? So we're spa?" They will return to their tables and continue in their prior mode. Or the professional will say, later, "This isn't doing what the book said it would for me. This has been a very costly mistake." *Becoming spa is a process, not a dictation, and must be approached as such in its implementation.*

WHERE ARE WE NOW?

The management team or professional must begin with *evaluating their present situation*, providing a full picture of the needs and possibilities. It should be done with a realistic view and open mind; the information is then used to plan for the ultimate goal. Evaluation will show the strengths and weaknesses of the current situation in relation to spa concept and enable more reliable planning in a purposeful march toward the goal. Mistakes will be fewer, and costs will be less.

The evaluation should include the menu, professional practices, home care and professional products, and the present physical layout and equipment. (see the relevant chapters) "Being spa" should be the underlying philosophy of these evaluations. Each evaluation must be done with this question in mind, "Does the client see this as spa concept?" (see Chapter 1.) Every decision must support this philosophy.

CHOOSING UPGRADES

After the evaluation, the management team or professional will know what areas need to be upgraded or redesigned. Plans for the process of change are completed before even one change or any announcement is made or the process will become cumbersome and confusing. There must be a "map" before leaving on the "trip," or the destination may never be reached!

The niche the salon serves must be confirmed and the ambiance to meet the needs and preferences of that niche verified or plans made for change toward them. The manicures and treatments are chosen, and the layout, equipment, and product needs are resourced to meet their needs (see Chapters 5 and 11).

The entrance routine is designed to fit the budget and staff (see Chapter 12). The manicures, treatments, programs, and packages must be chosen before the menu is designed.

The entry information materials are designed which takes time and should also be according to the budget and ambiance of the salon. Changes in the physical layout are determined, if needed, and the equipment is resourced.

Part of the choice of menu upgrades is the decision of "how much spa can we accomplish effectively and quickly?" and, "how much spa can we *afford* to implement right now?" Many potential spa concept salons and professionals may want to implement the new services slowly, one or two at a time. This is a valid approach to becoming spa concept and may be appropriate for many salons and professionals; sometimes "going for it all" can mean "going for failure," and implementation, one or two at a time, will be far better. Also, some clienteles respond better to a slower approach to services being added. Some professionals work better with this approach, and that is fine. Becoming spa is not supposed to be becoming stressed! Spa concept should be more relaxing for the professionals and clientele, not more stressful. The decision on how much spa can be introduced at once is for the evaluator to make and is an important consideration.

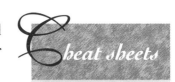

After a new manicure is chosen and the procedure is designed, a "Standard Practices Sheet" should be designed. A standard practices sheet is the new procedure, written out in full detail, to enable training of the manicuring staff. This sheet will:

• Reduce the time needed for training by reducing questions and confusion

• Maintain consistency of training

• Uphold accountability for consistent practices, over time

• "Pass on" procedures for new trainers and new employees

The sheet should be stored in a three-ring binder or such that contains copies of all the standard practice sheets for every skill being taught in the department.

A trainer must be responsible for keeping it up to date. Under no circumstances should it be allowed to become inaccurate or lack a procedure.

RESOURCING AND TESTING PRODUCTS AND EQUIPMENT

The professional products, equipment, and other needs should be resourced; specific criteria should be designed before the shopping to keep it focused and the choices narrow. For example, if the salon is searching for lotions, what is the net result a certain lotion must provide? Aromatherapy? High percentage alpha hydroxy acids? Low percentage? What price point should it be for the nail spa client? Be specific.

It is best that several products for each need should be evaluated and tested, then the choice made. Most importantly, the spa manicurists should be asked to test the available choices and express their thoughts on the products, because:

1. They are the ones who will work with the equipment and products.

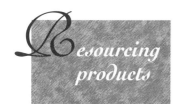

esourcing products

Several good resources are available in our industry are available through the trade magazines. Several of these magazines publish directories of the manufacturers yearly and they are free for the subscriber. These directories are worth the subscription investment for the searching resource person and are full of important information.

- *Nailpro Magazine* (The Gold Book)

- *Nails Magazine* (The Fact Book)

- *Skin Inc. Magazine* (The Directory)

- *American Salon* (The Green Book)

- *Modern Salon* (Focus 2000)

Aside from providing product resourcing information, the sponsoring magazines are educational resources that the spa manicurist should read thoroughly to support her skills, keep up with the trends, and stimulate her interest in her career. Growing professionals read their trade magazines.

2. They can put samples through paces that are relevant to the salon.

3. They are more experienced on these issues, usually, than the managers (unless, of course, the managers are in the specialty), and can at least provide valuable feedback.

4. Change is easier for professionals who have been a part of the process.

It is important all bases are covered on choices before the menu is designed and money is spent, and asking the professionals or a representative is an important aspect of that. One spa's experience with choosing equipment is an example. A day spa built a new location and custom designed a new pedicure station…without asking a pedicurist or manicurist for an opinion. It was beautiful, but the front of the tub was round and protruded toward the pedicurist. The result? The pedicurists working at those (very pretty) pedicure stations had to sit with their legs wide apart and lean far forward to get to their client's feet. The pedicure spas had to be replaced.

This same spa had a tiny closet for nail product storage, assuming the nail room would not need more. (It was one third the needed size.) There was no more space for expansion so the manicurists had to cope. There were many more details that would have been easier and less expensive to correct in the planning stage if a spa manicurist had been consulted.

Wise owners do not design or choose a piece of equipment, remodel or design a new location, choose products or the manicures for the menu without asking the opinion of a specialist who will work with them or a consultant who is experienced in the specialty.

EDUCATE, EDUCATE, EDUCATE

The decisions have been made and the decision-maker and consulting staff are happy with them. But, wait! The nail spa is not ready yet to launch the great new menu! The most important step is still to come: training. (Fig. 15–1)

The secret to full and successful implementation is *education for the professionals both in procedures and products before the implementation*. No professional will be sold on a procedure or product that she is not familiar with and confident in its results. If she is not, she will not offer either of them to clients. If she is not offering the new services and home care products to her clients, the process of upgrading to spa concept is a complete failure.

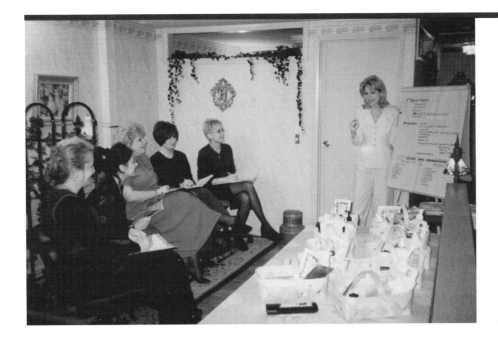

Figure 15-1

Training and educating professionals on products and procedures is the most important step.

Following are some of the subjects that would be included in the training of spa concept:

- *What is spa concept?* — Manicurists who understand and buy into the concept will be more productive and dedicated to the concept.

- *What's in it for me?* — Manicurists who understand how they will profit from spa concept will be more eager to make it successful.

- *Customer service* — Customer service in spa concept is more appropriately called 'client orientation' than customer service. The professionals will be dedicated to pampering and producing results and to meeting the needs of the client, not to performing a service.

- *Infection control* — A reminder of the basics with an explanation of how it is relevant to spa concept will be important.

- *Product knowledge and ingredient training* — Optimal results will be achieved by the spa manicurist who knows her products and how they will work for her clients. Home care products are only sold well by a knowledgeable professional.

- *Skin basics* — A manicurist who understands how products work on the skin will be able to explain how they work to their clients.

- *Analysis* — The very basis of success as a spa manicurist is the evaluation of the client and the recommendations that result from this thorough analysis.

Skin Analysis—The spa manicurist must understand what she will see and what to recommend that will more readily pamper and improve the client.

Nail Analysis—The client's nails will improve if the spa manicurist can correctly recommend appropriate nail treatments.

Service Recommendations—Regular clients will result if the spa manicurist is trained to recommend the appropriate manicures, programs, and packages to her client.

Home care training—Proper recommendations will extend the effects of the manicures and treatments and encourage the client to return for further care.

- *Technique training*—A spa manicurist must be confident and highly skilled in the manicures and treatments she recommends.

- *Reappointment/clientele building*—A spa manicurist must know how to ensure a regular clientele for herself and her salon.

- *Practice, practice, practice*—Practicing a technique until it is a routine for the professional ensures confidence, results, and clients who return.

Implementation is ready when all the changes are made, the products and equipment are in the salon, and training is complete. Now, put the new menu in place and go for it!

PERIODIC RE-EVALUATION/UPGRADING/RECONNECTION

The changes are made, and all is going well. Everyone can relax and usually enjoy being the only spa concept nail spa in town. There is one more step to design, however. Nail spas wishing to maintain spa concept must design a system for ensuring continued high quality and consistency in the procedures. The system must have these qualities:

- *Responsibility*—One person must be responsible for monitoring and dealing with complaints and problems. She will know that when a problem is repeated and it is a quality issue, retraining is indicated.

- *Accountability*—All professionals must be held accountable for the quality of their work. Those who recognized a need for retraining should be provided it on request; those who are assigned retraining due to a client problem must know it is appropriate.

- *Equipment*—The person responsible for monitoring quality is responsible for ensuring that all equipment is in excellent working order. The other manicurists will be responsible for using them correctly and keeping her informed.
- *Peer assistance*—Spa manicurists are eager to help each other if there is a skill problem so the spa and the professional get past it quickly. Help is the concept, not judgment or competition.
- *Training recheck*—Periodic meetings with the professionals for skill rechecks will keep the services consistent and of high quality. Spa manicurists should be trained to expect these sessions and welcome them, for their benefit and that of the salon.

If quality in a nail spa slips, it is usually because:

1. The original training was not adequate.
2. The quality assurance system has failed.
3. There is no effective focus on retraining.

A wise owner will know that client satisfaction revolves around quality care and that good training and follow-up go together with fewer complaints and higher client retention rates.

SKIN CARE FOR CLIENTS WITH ACRYLIC NAILS

Spa concept salons usually see their target clients as those who have natural nails. This focus is too narrow for the successful nail spa unless they have chosen natural nails as their niche point. The spa concept approach to client services is as important to the clients with acrylic nails as to those with natural nails. For that reason, spa manicuring should be implemented equally for both types of clients. After all, the only difference is that they wear enhancements.

If the trained and prepared spa manicurist trains her clients to see skin care recommendations as a part of their overall treatment, they will respond. She must strive to *educate* them to their need for skin care as support for their beautiful nails. They will love the extra pampering and appreciate the results of the treatments on their hands and arms.

Introducing Spa Treatments to the Existing Clients with Acrylics

Existing clients with acrylics may be hesitant to add the new treatments because the spa manicurist has not previously mentioned their skin care needs. On the other hand, they might be her most enthusiastic purchasers if they already trust her and are eager to have great skin.

The spa manicurist must be fully trained to do the new spa services on these clients before she offers them to her existing clientele. (Paying clients are not practice clients.) She must know the products, practice the services, and be ready to do them, knowing their benefits, their ingredients, and their results to answer clients' questions.

The spa manicurist can get her clients ready for the new services by being enthusiastic about the pending service during her training, study, and practice. She tells her clients about the new services each time they are in, building their interest. However, she should make them wait until she is fully prepared to provide the services, using this time to build an eagerness for the results the service will produce and an interest in booking the service. An example: "Janie, I've learned a great hydrating service for your hands that really works! I can't wait to do it on you!!! No, I can't do it on you yet. I'm still studying and taking classes on the whole system. You know, the structure of the skin, analysis, exfoliation products, all the things we have to know. And we're required to do a certain number on each other and the hair designers before we perform them on clients." Or, "I can't wait for you to see our new menu! You'll love it! It works! I'll let you know when I'm trained."

TIME AND PRICES

"How much time should this take?" and "How much should I charge?" are questions that can be answered only by the nail spa and the professionals performing the services. The criteria for the answers will be:

1. *The price* — Every service in a business must produce a certain amount per appointment book unit (usually 15 minutes). This amount, plus a fair profit, must be charged or the service must be eliminated.
2. *The spa manicurist's speed and expertise* — A manicurist must perform a high-quality service in a designated time or money and clients will be lost.
3. *The expectations of the clientele* — The expertise of the spa manicurists must meet the client's expectations in the time she wishes to spend and for the price she expects to spend.

4. The niche — It is a "maximum fit" situation. The highest amount the client will be willing to pay is charged, in turn with the least amount the salon can charge and make sufficient profit.

A wise owner will reach optimal productivity by designing a menu that meets the client's needs, resourcing and purchasing quality professional and home care products, hiring and training professionals to do quality services in a time that allows a good profit, and charging prices that allow the client to perceive them as a good value while providing the needed profit margin. Unity of these considerations will dictate the time and prices of services that the clients want to purchase.

IMPLEMENTING SPA SERVICES IN AN EXISTING SALON

Implementing spa services in a new nail spa is easy; the menu is designed, the products and equipment are purchased, the professionals are educated, and the clients are offered them when they first come to the salon. They have no expectations for that particular nail spa so they are open to suggestions.

Clients in an existing salon, however, are there as regulars because they like the status quo. They are more difficult to convince than the new ones who walk through the doors.

Existing clients do not like change. Even new services that will benefit them must be carefully introduced or they will fail miserably. The clients will need to be gently exposed to the salon's new upgraded manicures and their new improved results. Following are several methods for winning them over to the new services:

1. Sampling — Existing clients can be offered a free service to try a new service. However, many nail spas do not have the book space or professionals for this generosity. An alternate method is to have a drawing for new services. Each visit the client's name is entered for a free upgrade or manicure at her next visit. This will only work, however, if it is marketed heavily to the current clientele. Each week a different manicure or treatment can be offered, or a "blank check" can be offered for one of the new services her next visit. Every professional must discuss the manicure or treatment offered and the drawing with every client at her table, and let her see her name being entered. The promotional materials are designed well and abundant, not a little 8 x 10 handwritten sign over a plastic name-catcher bucket on the front desk.

2. *Rewards/thank yous* — Regular clients who are loyal to the nail spa can be offered a free upgrade to a new spa manicure or treatment as a thank you, unless time allows at this visit. She is told that she is being given the new service as a "thank you for your loyalty. We want you to know we appreciate you, and know you will like the new service." Clients love thank yous that are free and are open to reappointing for the service.

3. *Birthday and anniversary presents* — If the nail spa's client records have this information, a free upgrade, manicure, or treatment should be offered as a thank you present to loyal clients for their birthdays and anniversaries. The free services should be ones that are noted as a need during the client's analysis and should be thoroughly discussed concerning benefits to her hands.

4. *Suspense and delay* — This is the 'make them wait' discussed previously. Clients love new services that they are introduced to with a slow buildup of suspense and discussion.

5. *Package rewards* — Many spas are introducing maintenance packages, meaning a client who comes in for a regular manicure and pedicure, plus possibly a facial or a color appoints for a monthly appointment that includes all these in one visit. It saves both her and the spa time and the hassle of several visits. No discount is offered; the time savings is enough. This client can be rewarded for her loyalty by offering her a free upgrade in her manicure to one of the new services. It will introduce her to the new service and thank her for her loyalty at the same time.

6. *Two-for-one* — Some spas will offer a regular client a "two-for-one," which means the new manicure may accompany a pedicure, free at one visit. Some tie a two-for-one into her birthday or anniversary, sending her a coupon to bring a friend to enjoy her birthday visit with her or possibly her husband for her anniversary visit. A pampering service is introduced to her (and her friend or husband) as her present from "her" nail spa to her or to her husband or friend. They should be serviced beside each other at the same time, of course. A free sample of a lotion or oil with a bow on it, should be offered, also, with a full explanation of its use.

7. *Free upgrades* — The easiest introduction of a new service is through a free upgrade to a client's service. The enhanced results of the services will help the clients see the value in the upgraded services. If time permits, spa manicurists can incorporate one of the treatments into the standard service the client has been receiving regularly, at no charge or it can be offered with her next regular appointment. It gives the client a taste of what the new treatment is all about and tempts her for her next visit. Of course, it must be an appropriate upgrade, suggested through analysis, or it can be a pampering aromatherapy upgrade.

Introduction of the new manicures should be taken seriously in a salon. After the professionals and the nail spa are ready for implementation, a goal date should be set for every existing client to be introduced to the new manicures. Analysis should be done on every client, henceforth, and explanations should be complete as to the benefits of upgrading. If this is done, only a few clients will be booking the 'mini' in a short time and this will be a signal to cease offering it at all. New clients are offered only the new upgraded manicure.

No More Basic Manicures

After the new basic manicure has been accepted as the base manicure for a length of time and the water-soak manicure is merely a bad memory (aside from the exceptions), nail spas can step completely up to spa concept the same way. The spa manicure is offered to new clients and the new basic is removed from the menu, moving the basic up to spa manicure (see Chapter 5.) After all, the new basic, though it is the new skin care-based procedure, is not spa. It will not produce the results that a nail spa will wish for their clients due. (The cost difference here should not be high; this is still a basic manicure in time and effort. The differences are too subtle for a large difference in price.) Actually, most nail spa clients will slide into this manicure on their own, and soon the basic will be history, too.

Upgrading at the Nail Table

One of the inherent skills that a spa manicurist must develop is upgrading her clients to the services they need for their hand care. Again, hair designers and skin care specialists are trained in this skill; nail technicians do not. For that reason, it is a difficult skill to develop at the nail table without training, though it is an important skill to the success of the salon and the spa professional. Most important, however, it is important to the success of the professional's care for her clients. If she is not upgrading, she is not making the service suggestions that are necessary to meet her client's needs.

Some of the logical upgrades are:

- A new basic or spa manicure client comes in with hands that are showing a seasonal dryness; suggest a sloughing manicure to her for today, then a hydrating manicure for her next visit. The sloughing manicure is the same amount of time as her current appointment and will aid her by removing some of the dry surface cells. She should be sold a good emollient lotion and cuticle oil to get her hands on the road toward improvement.

- A client scheduled for a hydrating manicure sits down at the desk, sticks out her hands, and says, "I *need* this — I'm so stressed!" This client should be offered an aromatherapy manicure to aid her toward stress relief. The aromatherapy manicure takes the same amount of time as the hydrating manicure and she'll love it!

- A client is scheduled for a hydrating manicure and mentions the dark spots on her hands. Educate her concerning the causes for the spots (see Chapter 10) and suggest a glycolic series. Her manicure that day should be a sloughing treatment added to her hydrating manicure, and she should be sold the high percentage glycolic lotion to get her skin ready for the treatments. The sloughing treatment takes no more time within the hydrating manicure, and she will see immediate improvement that will be supported by the lotion.

Every client has further needs that a trained and product knowledgeable spa manicure professional can see and recommend. However, a wise professional only makes service suggestions that are supported by what she sees as needs the client has. Suggestions are made during analysis, before the care of the service begins, and supported throughout the service through the points.

Successful implementation of spa concept in a nail salon is a process that involves methodical planning, decision-making, and professional focus. These will be tedious at times, fun at other times, and agonizing at others. Once done, however, the nail salon is no longer a salon. *Now it's a nail spa!*

Spa Manicuring for the Salon and Spa

The Decision and Implementation of Spa Manicure

Linda Champion, Golden Shears, Runnemede, NJ
"Best in South Jersey—Manicures" Courier Post, Cherry Hill, NJ,
"Readers Choice Awards, 1999"

In October 1998, I attended the "Nail Those Profits At Sea" cruise. The cruises are both fun and learning, so I attended a Spa Manicuring Class, taught by Janet McCormick. I was only slightly interested in learning about new manicure techniques since about 90 percent of our clients have acrylic nails, but I decided to sit through the class, figuring I'd probably get something out of it.

Just a few minutes into the class, wheels began to turn in my head. Why not upgrade our nail "department" to spa-level? "The Nail Spa at Golden Shears" sounded so professional. I sat in the class wishing the staff members were listening with me to hear these new options in servicing their clients. Our world was expanding before my eyes beyond just doing an awesome fingernail.

When I arrived home, I reviewed our current service menu...the one that I once thought was impressive and professional. Now I saw a basic group of services with hardly anything stimulating or different to entice clients to try a new service. Also, it lacked the feeling of relaxation, the tone of wellness and luxury that the popular new spa treatments can do for the mind, body, and spirit. I wanted this for our clients, and for the technicians!

Still, our clientele was 90 percent acrylics. How was I ever going to promote all these new manicures? Why would I even want to tempt my loyal acrylic clients to "go natural" just to reap the benefits of spa treatments? Then I realized, that was exactly it—*treatments*. Acrylic clients can also benefit from spa hand treatments, without getting the full manicures. For instance, we could offer the Salt Glow Treatment, alone or with the acrylic service to the acrylic clients, and they could reap the same benefits as the spa manicure clients do on their skin. We could do any spa service before or after her fill. I decided to check this out. I called Janet with some basic questions and got started.

continued

Planning

Now it was time to go shopping. Janet had recommended many types of skin products in the class that I hadn't heard of before. She taught us how to read ingredients, look them up if need be, what to look for in them, and much more. The shopping, with that information in my possession, was fun. First, I selected a full spectrum of spa "treatment" products, and resourced the support products that were needed to perform them well. I ordered professional and home care sizes, and design a great home care display area. The difficult part was the need to be educated in areas I'd never imagined, such as aromatherapy, alpha hydroxy acids, emollients, exfoliates, minerals, vitamins, and more, but I began to love learning this stuff! Soon I was addicted and wanted to learn more and more.

While I was doing all my homework, I kept it under my hat for fear of losing the manicurists' focus if resourcing dragged out into too much time. Then, I called a staff meeting and introduced them to the world of "spa" using my notes from the cruise. The technicians were excited! But this class was only the first step to pulling this off effectively. Two weeks later we brought in Janet. We had our first day-long class, and they joined me in the knowledge of "being spa." We learned analysis, the treatments, recommending, and manicures. Later, after practicing the skills, we had another day of performing the treatments to aid us in being focused on the correct methods, and practiced analysis mechanics.

Implementation

After a third and final practice class, we held an "Employee Appreciation Night" to pamper the other salon personnel with our new services. With experiencing the various spa treatments, they too became excited to introduce them to their clients. We found it a great way to involve the entire salon in spa concept.

We weren't finished yet. Now we were ready for "Client Appreciation Day." We sent an invitation to our clients (in letter form) to invite them to come in on a particular day to learn more about our new spa treatments, experience the luxury and learn about the

continued

underlying beauty and health they provide. I explained how home care is necessary to expand the life of these services, and that we now have the professional products to "meet their needs." The day was a great success, and the clients eagerly added the new treatments to their future appointments. Now, we perform analysis on every client, acrylic or not, and routinely make recommendations for treatments, manicures, and home care. They expect them and appreciate the improvements the spa services produce for their skin. The launch of spa concept was successful!

Since our "nail department" became a "nail spa," we have a whole new view of "doing nails." Our vision has been expanded from just the nail plate to the entire hand, arm, and elbow, and from the toes to the feet, legs, and knees. "Being spa" has opened a whole new world for The Nail Spa at Golden Shears. And we love it.

EPILOGUE SPA CONCEPT: AN ATTITUDE

Being spa is an attitude, not a place (see Chapter 1); it is an *orientation*, an *awareness*, a *professionalism* being provided for the client at a particular level of service. Spa concept professionals will nurture the development of this attitude in every aspect of their salon life and carry it over into their personal advocacy of the salon and their peers; they will promote the salon when off duty as a great place to work and a great place to be, and they will promote their salon peers as quality professionals and great people to work with.

Spa manicuring techniques and the accompanying attitudes are integral to achieving spa concept within a nail spa. Spa manicuring techniques bring spa concept *to the nail table*. It redefines the care of the client, expanding treatment from the client's nail plate only, to treating the full area of the manicurist's license: the nail plate, cuticles, hands, arms, and elbows of the clients. A manicurist who integrates spa concept into her professional life will gain a new attitude toward her work. She will:

- *Develop new decision-making skills reflecting spa concept in her minute-by-minute, day-by-day, and career life.* She will ask herself, "What is the spa concept decision here?" knowing that will be the right thing to do. For example, when deciding on a client treatment, she will consciously say to herself, "What does this client need today and next time she comes in?" When tempted to discuss a personal issue in the spa, she will stop and think to herself, "This should wait until we are in the lounge or out of the client's treatment area." She will subconsciously know if an activity is or is not what a spa client would want to experience.

- *Direct her professional activities toward client orientation.* She will connect her potential for success with that of enabling the client's enjoyment and rejuvenation.

- *Develop a supportive attitude toward the success of the salon and her peers.* She will connect her potential for success with that of the salon and her peers.

- *Develop new expectations for her performance and that of her peers.* A spa manicurist sets a high level of expectations of performance for herself, and she expects her peers to also meet these high expectations.

- *Continually develop her professional skills and work-life toward being spa.* This professional will seek out training and constantly look toward defining/redefining the salon services and her skills toward achieving spa concept (see Chapter 1).

As a result of spa concept, this professional will be more confident and successful, gain satisfaction from her work, and reach her career potentials. Her salon will be a great place to work in the midst of achieving high success, and clients will line up to spend their money in an ambiance or relaxation and rejuvenation. *It will be spa.*

REFERENCES

1. Popcorn, F. (1991) The Popcorn Report, (New York: Doubleday).

2. Scher, R.K., & D.C., III. (1990). Nails, therapy, diagnosis, surgery. Philadelphia: Saunders.

3. Satur, N.M. (1996, April). Formaldehyde fears, Nailpro Magazine, p.67

4. Seiling, J. (1997). The membership organization: Achieving top performance through the new workplace community. (Palo Alto, CA). Davies Black Publications.